YOUR GUIDE TO HIGH BLOOD PRESSURE CONTROL

MARTIN HAGLUND

CONTENTS

INTRODUCTION

After more than 10 years of high blood pressure I decided to take some action. At that point in life I was on three different drugs to control the pressure and suffering from frequent and massive headaches. I decided to look for a way to normalize my blood pressure without medication. I didn't want any quick fixes, or extreme life style changes. It would have to be something I could live with in the long run without changing my way of living dramatically, and the measures taken would have to be low budget. So I launched my project focusing on diet and simple physical activity.

1 THE PROJECT

Although I had some ideas about healthy food and physical activity, I needed to do some research on these subjects, and their influence on blood pressure.

I discovered DASH (Dietary Approaches to Stop Hypertension), and found a lot of information about the issues I was looking for. According to DASH, high blood pressure can be prevented—and lowered—if you take these steps:

- Follow a healthy eating plan, such as DASH, that includes foods lower in salt and sodium.
- Maintain a healthy weight.
- Be moderately physically active for at least 30 minutes on most days of the week.
- If you drink alcoholic beverages, do so in moderation.

If you already have high blood pressure, and your doctor has prescribed medicine, take your medicine, as directed, and also follow these steps. I have been through scores of other sources of info, and they pretty much give the same advice.

Blood pressure is affected by several factors. I needed to know which, and my baseline score on these to be able to measure any progress on my way to the goal.

1.1 RISK FACTOR BASELINE

OVERWEIGHT

According to DASH - Being overweight or obese increases your risk of developing high blood pressure. In fact, your blood pressure rises as your body weight increases. Losing even 10 pounds can lower your blood pressure - and losing weight has the biggest effect on those who are overweight and already have hypertension. My baseline weight was 275 lbs (125 kg).

Two key measures are used to determine if someone is overweight or obese. These are body mass index, or BMI, and waist circumference.

BMI is a measure of your weight relative to your height. It gives an approximation of total body fat - and that's what increases the risk of diseases that are related to being overweight. My BMI was more than 33.

But BMI alone does not determine risk. For example, in someone who is very muscular or who has swelling from fluid retention (called edema), BMI may overestimate body fat. BMI may underestimate body fat in older persons or those losing muscle.

That's why waist measurement is often checked as well. Another reason is that too much body fat in the stomach area also increases disease risk. A waist measurement of more than 35 inches in women and more than 40 inches in men is considered high. My waistline was 47 inches (117 cm).

SMOKING

I don't smoke or use tobacco in any way. I used to be a "party smoker" a few years ago, but now this risk factor is eliminated.

ALCOHOL

More than moderate, but not excessive consumption of mostly wine and beer, and occasionally a few drinks.

PHYSICAL INACTIVITY

For many years I tried to do some workouts 2-4 times each week, depending on my travelling schedule. At the time the project started I had too long breaks from my physical activity – there could be weeks and months without any activity except the Sunday walk. The time periods I was inactive had been longer and longer the years before.

WORK

My excuse for not being physically active was my work schedule. My job required a lot of travelling, combined with irregular and sometimes long working days. I also lacked the discipline I needed to use the available time I had now and then to do some exercises.

MEDICATION

When I started the project I was on three different medicines for controlling my high blood pressure.

1.2 GOALS

My overall goal was a normal blood pressure without medication.

To reach the main goal I focused on some partial goals

	Baseline	Goal
Weight	275 lbs	<230 lbs
BMI	33	<30
Waistline	47 inches	<40 inches

To reach these goals I needed to

- be physically more active – min 30 minutes a day
- eat more healthy food
- burn more energy than I consumed

1.3 KEY SUCCESS FACTORS

To get the project going I soon realized that I needed to pay attention to a few issues.

I know my weaknesses and I knew that concerning the food and the exercising there had to be

- Easy access — I wanted to find the food in ordinary grocery stores, and I wanted to start the workouts from home
- Minimum preparation time — the food should be easy and fast, and the workouts should be possible to start without a lot of preparation

This made it easier to follow the eating and exercise plans.

PLANNING

First thing about eating healthy food is that it's available when you are hungry. So I needed to plan a few days ahead when I was shopping groceries.

PREPARATION

If you have built up motivation for doing some activity – except for your everyday activities like cleaning or gardening or walk to your work place - there's two important issues to consider:

- You should know what workout to do
- You need the gear and equipment to do it

I planned my workouts for each week, and I always had the necessary gear available.

CHANGE YOUR MINDSET

It helped me a lot to change the way I was thinking about some activities I used to dislike – like carwash, cleaning, gardening and other similar activities.

When the house looked messy or the lawn needed some work, I used to call someone. Today I look upon it as a way to fulfill my goal of doing 30-60 minutes of physical activity each day. And I even save some money!

Don't make it a project

I know I called this a project. But the thing about a project is that it comes to an end if it's successful. For me it was important that I could live with the changes I was planning to do, and turn it into my normal life style. One way to think about this was "gradual change" – don't turn everything around overnight.

That's why I searched for food and activities that was affordable, easy accessible and easy to implement in my daily routines.

1.4 IMPLEMENTATION

How did I go about it? I focused on two main issues:

- Diet – chapter 2 describes the main ingredients in my diet. I did – and do - eat a lot of other stuff, but I ensured that I consumed most of these foods on a regular basis
- Physical activity – chapter 3 shows my favorite workouts, and the backbone of the physical side of the project.

In addition to eating more healthy food I also gradually reduced the amount of food in each serving.

After a few months I introduced (to myself) the 30MAD (30 Minutes-A-Day) concept:

Each day should contain at least 30 minutes of activity. So I started doing some simple physical exercises on the days I didn't do my regular workouts.

1.5 RESULTS

It took three years to reach my goal. A more disciplined person than me could do this in a shorter time, I'm sure, but better late than never.

The challenge now is to keep going like this.

The food issue is no problem. I buy, eat and like this kind of food – and try to keep the volume down in each meal.

The physical activity part requires a lot more attitude. I need to work with myself to stay motivated and focused.

2. FOOD

According to "Your Guide to Lowering Blood Pressure with DASH":

What you eat affects your chances of getting high blood pressure.

And more:

A healthy eating plan can both reduce the risk of developing high blood pressure and lower a blood pressure that is already too high.

I studied carefully the information in DASH, which stands for "Dietary Approaches to Stop Hypertension." It says you can reduce your blood pressure by eating foods that are low in saturated fat, total fat, and cholesterol, and high in fruits, vegetables, and low-fat dairy foods. The DASH eating plan includes whole grains, poultry, fish, and nuts, and has low amounts of fats, red meats, sweets, and sugared beverages. It is also high in potassium, calcium, and magnesium, as well as protein and fiber. Eating foods lower in salt and sodium also can reduce blood pressure.

The DASH eating plan has more daily servings of fruits, vegetables, and grains than you may be used to eating. Those foods are high in fiber, and eating more of them may temporarily cause bloating and diarrhea. To get used to the DASH eating plan, gradually increase your servings of fruits, vegetables, and grains.

In addition to the DASH recommendations, I did some research myself, and got some advice and help from other sources. This chapter present some of the foods considered most healthy.

2.1 MOST HEALTHY FOOD

My everyday diet is very much concentrated on some of the foods described here. This is very much easy accessible, affordable food and considered very healthy. I have added some comments on their influence on blood pressure and healthy heart.

I don't eat all of these all the time. A few of them is taken on a daily basis, others are more irregular. And of course I eat other things as well – like too much pasta.

Avocado

The avocado used to be considered a "fatty" food, and doctors recommended eating fewer of them. Recent research has shown that the avocado actually has many health benefits and is one of the healthiest foods you can eat.

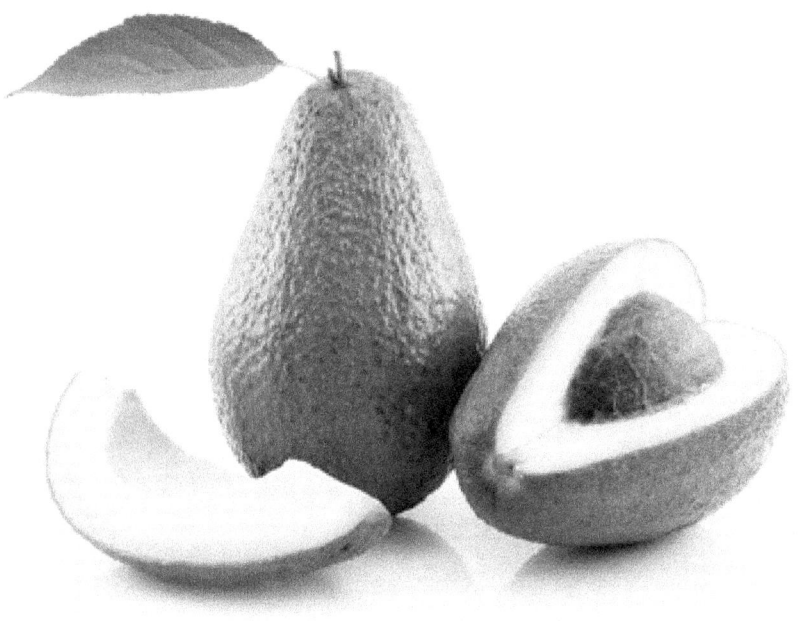

Avocados are particularly helpful in preventing cardiovascular problems, when you eat 1/6 of one per day.

The Center for Disease Control recommends replacing other fats in your diet with monounsaturated fats, like avocado, or polyunsaturated ones. All fats are not bad for you. Vitamins A, D, E and K, are fat-soluble, and without fats, your body can't absorb them. A recent review of research found that people who eat very low fat diets are at greater risk for heart disease.

The monounsaturated fat in avocados increases the level of HDL (good cholesterol) by 11% and lowers the level of bad cholesterol. High levels of "bad" cholesterol (LDL) increase risk for heart disease, but a healthy diet can help control it.

Avocados contain 20 nutrients, including a high level of potassium, which helps to control high blood pressure. When blood pressure is high, it increases the risk of a heart attack.

The vitamin B6 and folic acid in avocados regulate your body's level of homocysteine; when levels are too high, there is greater risk of heart disease. Other nutrients include glutathione vitamin E, and oleic acid, an omega-9 fatty acid.

FAT-FREE MILK

Dairy products are part of a healthy diet, adding the calcium and proteins needed for growing bones and teeth and giving energy. However, dairy products are also very high in saturated fats.

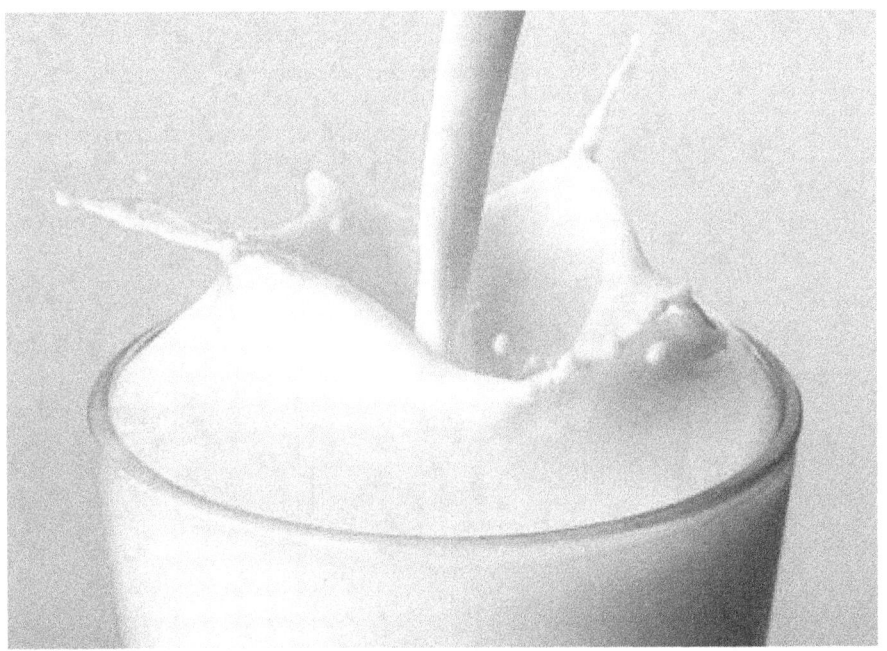

The Center for Disease Control says saturated fats increase risk of coronary heart disease and should only be 10% of our total diet. Fats don't directly raise blood pressure, they do cause weight gain, which increases risk of high blood pressure.

Whole milk contains between 62-70% saturated fat, while beef contains only 38-49% - but skim milk has no fat at all. The American Heart Association recommends that you drink fat-free milk, which cuts down on saturated fats, and also lowers your risk of stroke.

When you take all the fat out of milk, you also lose the fat-soluble vitamins, so skim milk is fortified with vitamin D, which enables the body to process the calcium in it. The vitamins added equal what was lost with the fat. An 8-oz. glass of milk has 30% of the calcium and 32% of the vitamin D you need daily.

Salmon

Experts seem to agree that salmon is among the very best foods for a healthy heart. It's high in protein and in the omega-3 fatty acids that promote heart health. The omega-3 fatty acids also keep blood pressure lower.

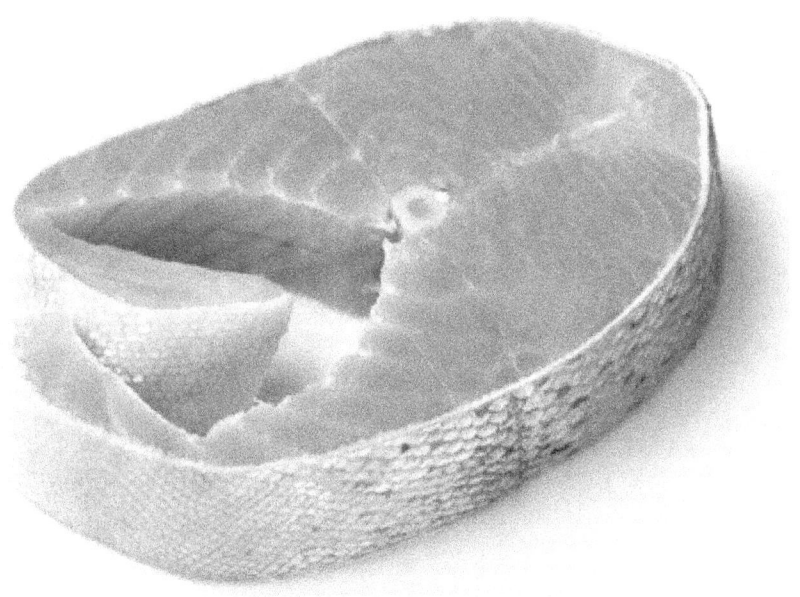

According to the American Heart Association, you should eat salmon, or other oily fish like lake trout or albacore tuna, at least two times a week. They also say that salmon has two omega-3 fatty acids that are particularly good for people who are already at risk for heart disease. Salmon is also high in beneficial micronutrients.

Wild vs. Farmed

There's a lot of controversy regarding the difference between wild salmon and farmed salmon. Some experts say we should avoid farmed salmon because of the contaminants in fish farms. Dr. Dariush Mozzafarian of the Harvard School of Public Health said that the cardiac benefits of eating salmon are between 100 and 400 times greater than the health risks of contaminants, and "It's much more dangerous not to eat the salmon."

Eggs

The egg's reputation suffered in the past because of anxiety about cholesterol, but recent research has good news for egg fans: dietary cholesterol is not a factor in getting heart disease for most people.

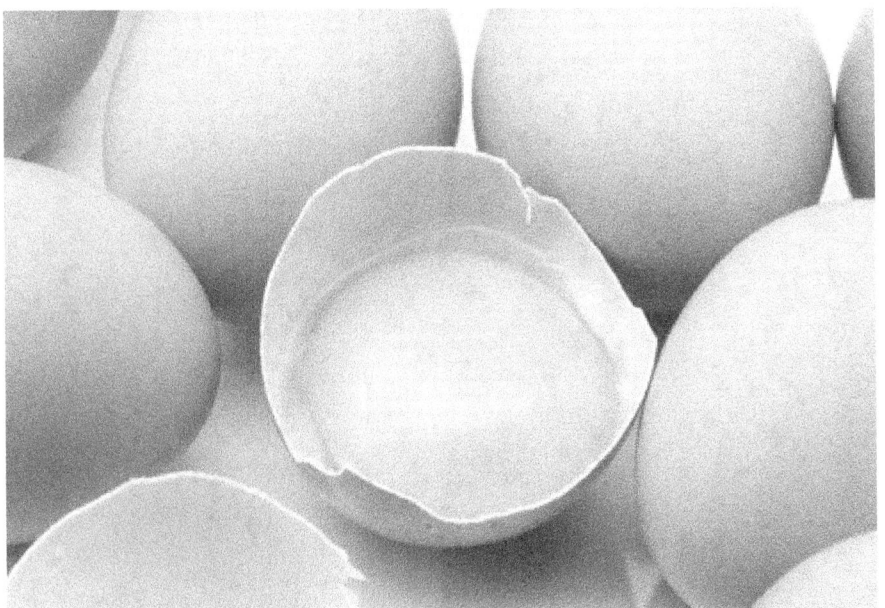

Eggs are a rich source of amino acids, riboflavin, and selenium and they contain plenty of protein. At only 70 calories per whole egg, they provide energy and a satisfied feeling that curbs hunger longer, and we eat less at the next meal.

All the worrisome fat and cholesterol in eggs is in the yolk, but egg whites are a very heart healthy protein. The American Heart Association recommends limiting our daily cholesterol intake to 300 mg per day, but an egg with its yolk has 185 mg. Most doctors are saying an egg a day is fine for most diets, and eggs without yolks are among the healthiest foods, with only 17 calories in each white.

GREEK YOGURT

Yogurt made in the traditional Greek way drains the whey from the solids. The result is a denser, creamier product with twice the protein of American style products, and a tangy flavor.

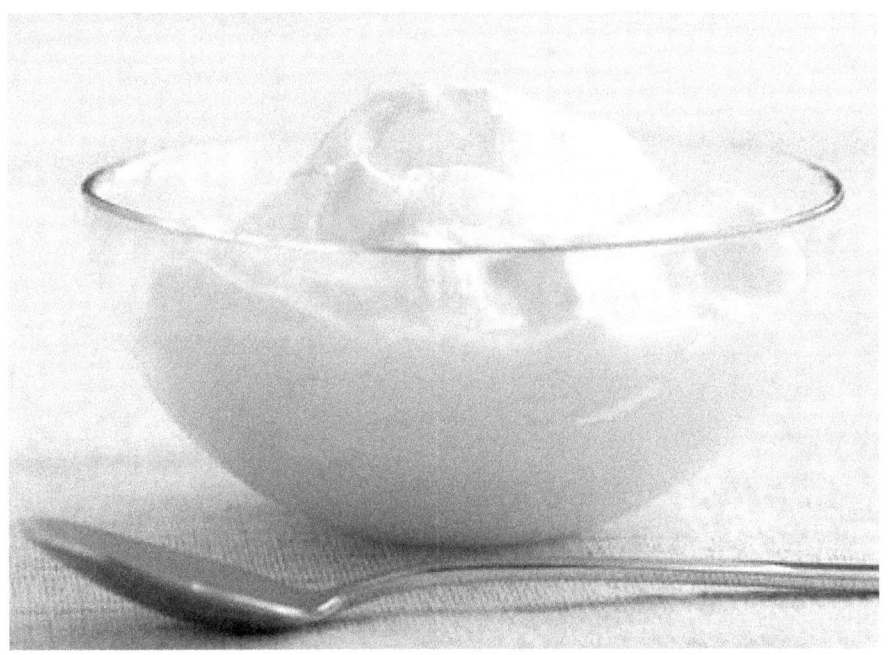

Besides being high protein, it has a wealth of vitamins and minerals - phosphorous, riboflavin, zinc, iodine, pantothenic acid (vitamin B5), vitamin B12, and calcium.

Yogurt from Greece also contains a higher percentage of omega-3 fatty acids because of the native plants, grasses, and shrubs in diets of sheep and cattle.

The American Journal of Clinical Nutrition published a study showing that eating Greek yogurt can reduce your risk of having high blood pressure. The high potassium content is believed to shed excess sodium from the body, and too much salt is known to contribute to the risk of high blood pressure. Participants in the study who ate two (or more) helpings of low-fat yogurt and other dairy products a day had 54% lower rates of high blood pressure than participants who ate the less or none.

A study at the University of Knoxville, Tennessee, showed that eating yogurt helps you lose weight, too. Lead researcher Michael Zemel says that yogurt's high calcium content sends messages to fat cells on your belly that produce cortisol, a hormone that encourages your body to add fat, telling them to stop producing so much cortisol. People in this study who ate yogurt lost 22% more weight.

Beans

Beans are one of the healthiest foods you can eat, and perhaps one of the very cheapest.

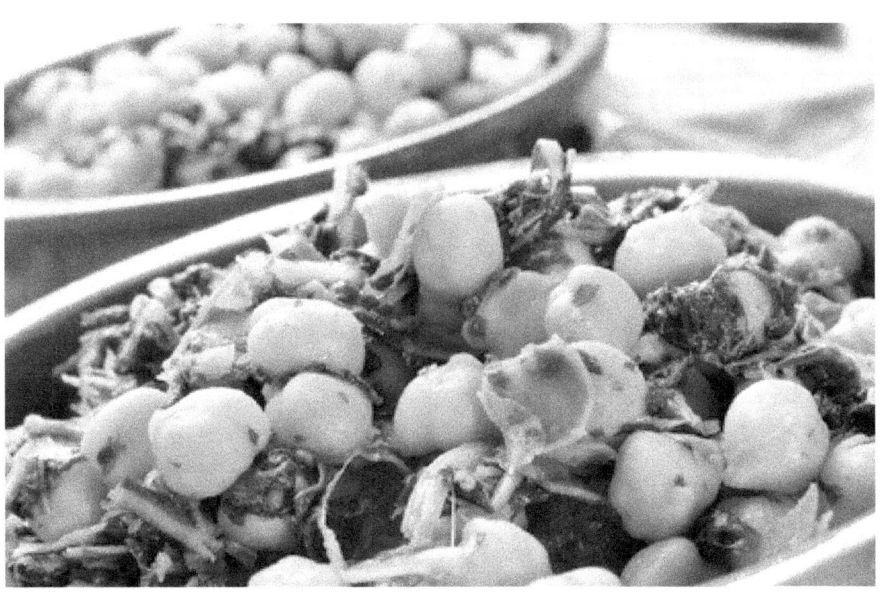

Dried beans, soaked and cooked slowly over low heat, have abundant fiber, potassium, magnesium, calcium, iron, copper, phosphorus, folic acid, a-linolenic acid - a known preventative for cardiovascular diseases - and plenty of protein. They offer reduced risk of stroke or high blood pressure, thanks to the high potassium content.

In a 2005 study, researchers at the Harvard School of Public Health determined that people who ate a half-cup serving of cooked dried beans four times a week showed a lower incidence of heart disease, and cited another study which found a 22% lower rate among participants who ate beans frequently. They also point out that the complex carbohydrates in beans reduce the glycemic load, and are helpful for weight loss. Eating beans twice a day isn't necessary to get the benefits.

Lean Beef

There's little question that the fast-food burger a day does not promote a healthy heart. However, lean beef can be a beneficial part of your diet, as it contains important micronutrients like iron, zinc, and B-vitamins, and a significant amount of protein.

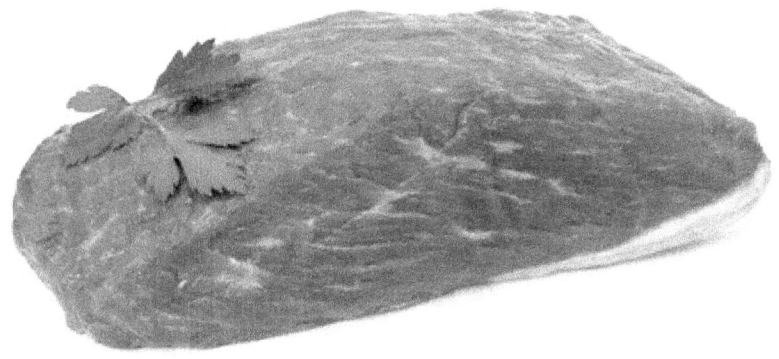

The Mayo Clinic suggests eating it in moderation – occasionally - and choosing cuts of meat that are low in fat. They recommend lean cuts that have no more than 10 grams of fat in a 3.5 ounce serving, with 4.5 grams of saturated fat, or extra lean cuts with only 5 grams of fat, 2.5 of them saturated.

A total of twenty-nine different cuts of meat have been identified as meeting the nutritional standards for lean. Mayo Clinic researchers recommend top, bottom, or eye of round, steaks or roasts, sirloin tip side steaks, or top sirloin steak.

Not all beef is the same. Dr. Martha Grogan, at the Mayo Clinic, points out that grass-fed beef may have some heart benefits that you won't find in factory farms cattle. Grass-fed cows can produce leaner meat, higher amounts of omega-3 fatty acids, and more conjugated linoleic acids, fats believed to reduce heart disease.

GARLIC

Garlic is one of those wonder foods that is both a delicious addition to the food we eat and also highly medicinal. It's a powerhouse of phyto-nutrients, antioxidants, minerals, and vitamins. Vitamin B6, vitamin C, iron, copper, calcium, manganese, potassium, zinc, iron, magnesium, and selenium - an important part of heart health - make this herb a valuable addition to a diet of the healthiest foods.

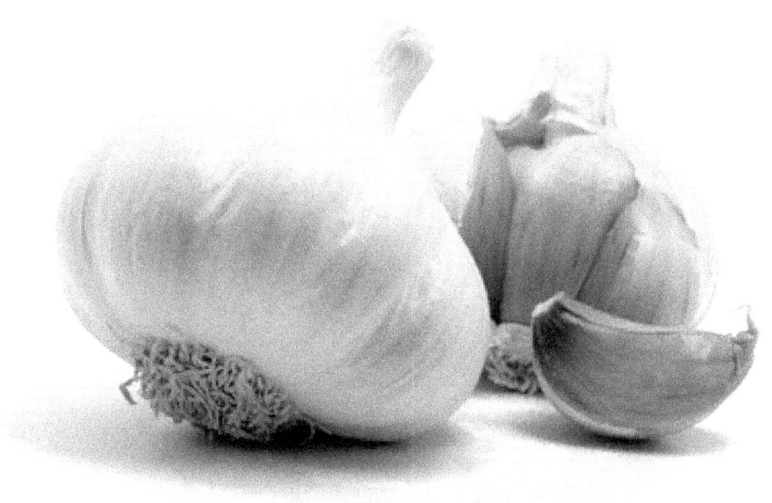

If you don't like the flavor, you can take it in capsule form, although eating the food itself is thought to be more beneficial.

Doctors are now recommending taking garlic extract capsules to treat high blood pressure. According to the experts on WebMD, you should take between 200 and 400 mg three times a day, but advise that eating a fresh clove once a day can also be beneficial. Cutting or crushing garlic releases an enzymatic chain reaction to produce allicin, which reduces the stiffness in blood vessels, and lowers your blood pressure.

The compounds in garlic reduce the coronary artery disease risks and stroke. Its high selenium content prevents formation of platelets, as well as providing a co-factor in the release of antioxidants in the body. Given the amount of garlic used in Mediterranean cooking, it's no surprise that people in that part of the world have a very low incidence of heart disease.

Nuts

Nuts are often overlooked as a regular staple of your diet, but their contribution to a healthy heart is very significant. Loaded with protein, anti-oxidants, Omega-3 fatty acids, high vitamin content, and monosaturated fats that lower bad cholesterol, they're one of the healthiest foods you can eat.

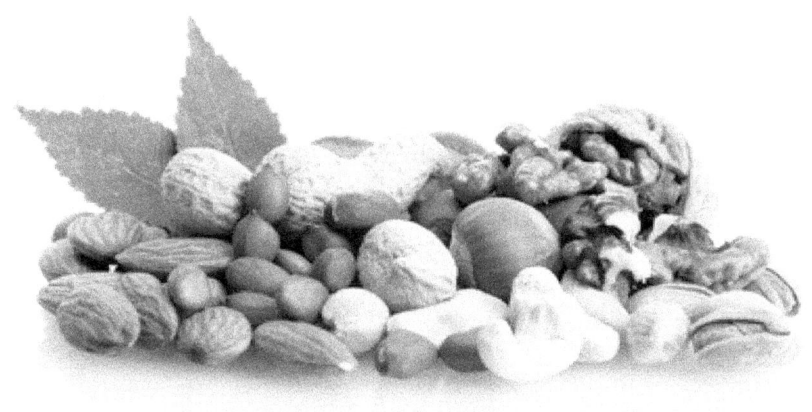

Dr. Emilio Ros of the Endocrinology and Nutrition Service in Barcelona wrote that, "Diet changes remain the cornerstone for prevention and treatment of CVD, and the emerging picture is that nut consumption beneficially influences cardiovascular risk." The DASH diet (Dietary Approaches to Stop Hypertension) suggests eating between 4 and 5 one-ounce servings of nuts, seeds, and beans every week to lower blood pressure.

Each variety of nuts has different healthful properties. Almonds have more fiber than other nuts, and are highest in vitamin E. Macadamia and hazelnuts have the highest amounts of monosaturated fats, and although hazelnuts have a higher total fat content than other nuts, they're also very high in potassium and magnesium. Walnuts contain more antioxidants than any other kind of nut, and researchers believe that they protect against the cellular damage that causes heart disease. Pecans help prevent the formation of plaque in arteries, and they also are very high in antioxidants. Pistachios, very low in sodium, are rich in potassium, which increases healthy blood pressure.

Oatmeal

This is clearly one of the healthiest foods you can eat. It's high in fiber, and researchers are saying that fiber attaches to cholesterol and flushes it out of your body.

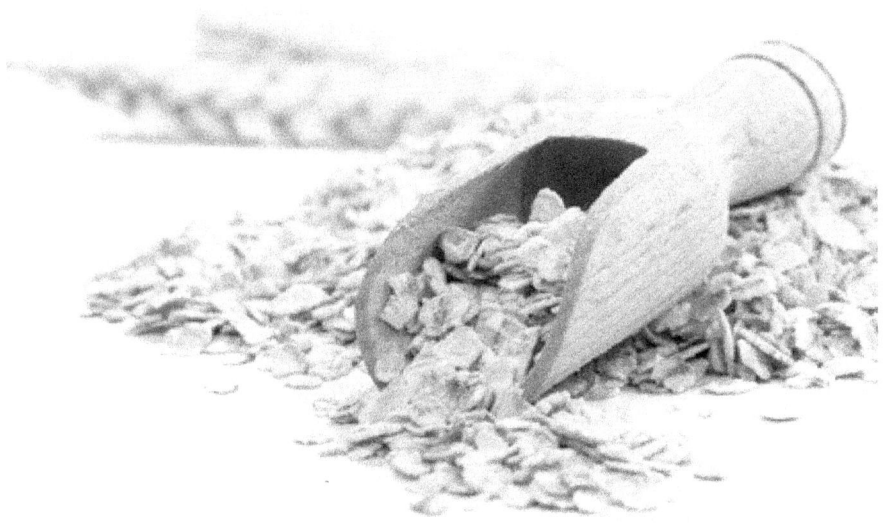

A study published in the American Journal of Clinical Nutrition tested the effects of a high fiber cholesterol-lowering diet and the effects of taking medications to control it, and found that the results were the same. And the soluble fiber in oatmeal is recommended by the American Journal of Lifestyle

Medicine because it "contains properties that bolster cardiovascular health."

The fiber in oatmeal contains a substance called beta-glucan. The journal Vascular Health Risk Management concluded that beta-glucans can "alleviate ischemic heart injury." Oatmeal also has significant mineral content: a cup of it has 25% of the magnesium you need in a day, 30% of the phosphorus, 10% of the iron, and a good amount of manganese, copper, and selenium; plus 5 grams of protein.

If you have high blood pressure, eating oatmeal can keep it down. According to the American Dietetic Association, a study showed that people with high levels of cholesterol and blood pressure were able to lower blood pressure by incorporating whole grains like oatmeal in their diets.

FLAXSEED

While flaxseed isn't one of those things you might want to make a meal of, it is a remarkably healthy addition to the other foods you eat. It contains a significant dose of soluble fiber, helpful in maintaining healthy digestion, and it's believed to be useful in lowering levels of bad cholesterol.

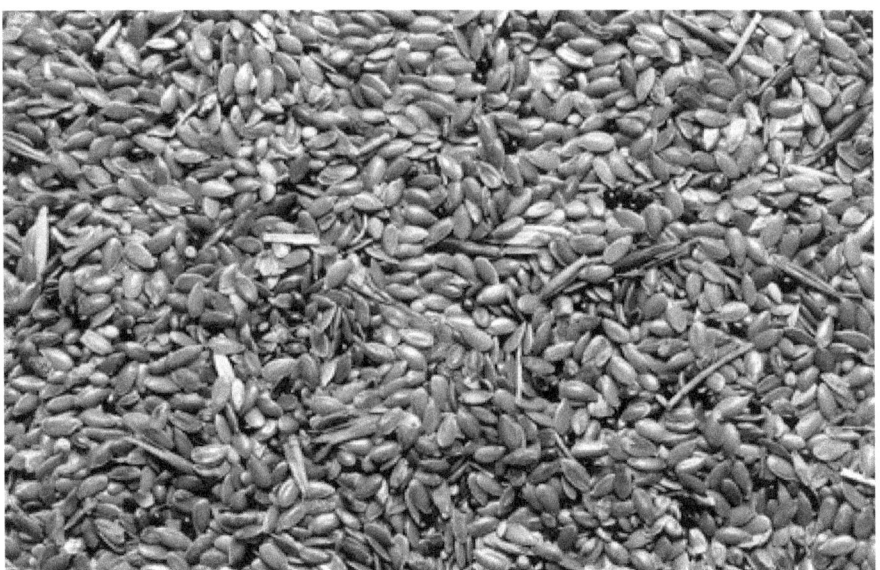

Flaxseed is full of plant-based omega-3s that keep arteries from hardening, maintain the steady rhythm of your heart, and stop platelets from building up. One researcher found that the lingans in flaxseed reduce the concentration of plaque in your arteries as much as 75%. Other research is showing that the amino acids in flaxseed help get your blood pressure down, and it also has anti-inflammatory benefits. Flaxseed is getting more attention from researchers now, as recent studies have shown that it may have a lot to offer.

Consult your doctor if you are planning to take a flaxseed supplement. It should not be taken when you are taking other medications orally. Also, because of its effect on digestion, it can alter how your body processes food, and can result in constipation or diarrhea.

Olive Oil

The oil cold-pressed from olives (virgin) is the jewel of the Mediterranean diet, and a great substitute for other fats in your diet. Loaded with vitamins E and K, with a very high antioxidant content, this oil offers numerous benefits to your health. Low in saturated fats, and high in monounsaturated ones, it lowers bad cholesterol and increases the good kind.

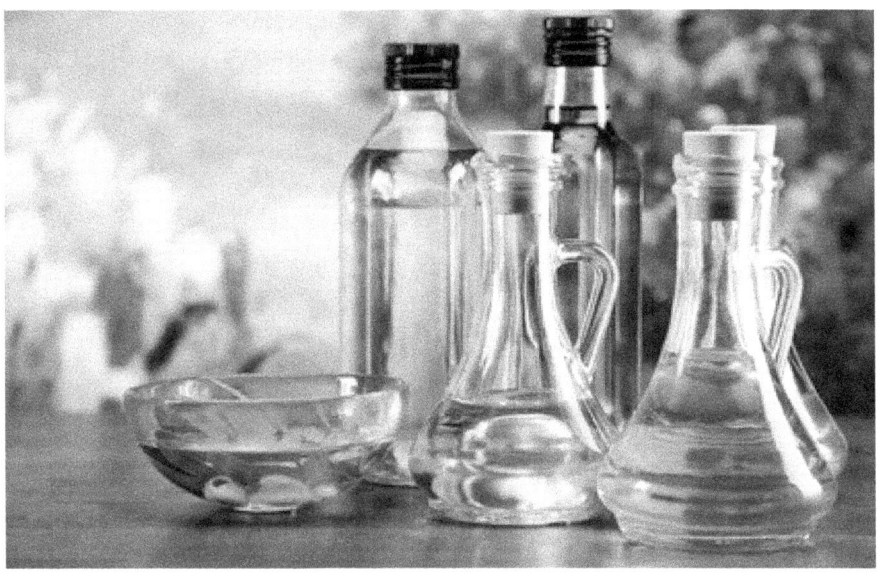

The phenolic compounds in olive oil, such as the potent anti-oxidants oleuropein and oleocanthal, have anti-inflammatory properties beneficial to heart health. It's no surprise the Mediterranean countries where olive oil is the principle source of fat in the diet, also have the lowest rates of coronary heart disease. The plant sterols in olive oil, according to the FDA, "may reduce the risk of heart disease."

While olive oil provides numerous benefits to your health, it is best to incorporate it in cooking and not just have some as an addition to your diet. A tablespoon of this oil has about 120 calories, so you would want to use it as a salad dressing, or to flavor vegetables like broccoli, rather than thinking of it as a potential dietary supplement. A tablespoon a day provides the benefits and turns healthy food into the healthiest food you can eat.

Broccoli

There aren't enough great things to say about broccoli. A one cup serving gives you 200% of your daily requirement of vitamin C, as much calcium as 4 ounces of milk, almost 1100 IUs of vitamin A, and healthy doses of vitamins B1, B2, B3, B6, beta-carotene, iron, magnesium, potassium, iron, and zinc. It also has some omega-3 fatty acids and antioxidant content.

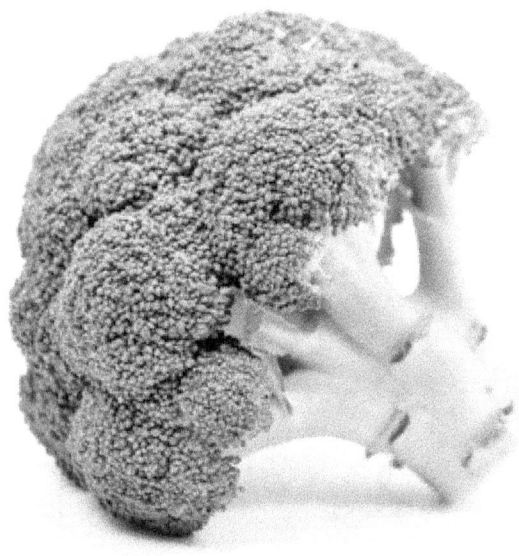

Very low in calories, a medium stalk of broccoli has 16% of the fiber you need daily. It's an invaluable addition to your diet.

The indoles in broccoli are phytochemicals that detoxify your body and are useful in prevention of high blood pressure and heart disease. Dr. Peter Hoagland and Dr. Philip Pfeffer for the USDA's research center in Philadelphia found that a fiber in broccoli, calcium pectate, enables the liver to retain cholesterol in your liver, rather than releasing it into your bloodstream, and they "found broccoli equally as effective as some cholesterol lowering drugs."

Spinach

The health benefits of leafy green vegetables are well known, and spinach is among the very best. It has plenty of fiber, protein, the anti-oxidant benefits of plentiful vitamin A, plus B2, B6, C, E, and K. It's also rich in phosphorus, niacin, zinc, selenium, manganese, magnesium, iron, copper, folates, and omega-3 fatty acids.

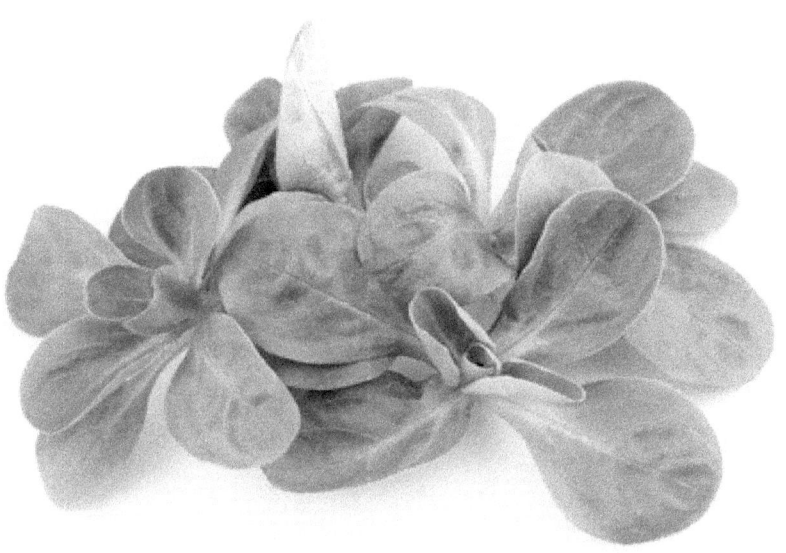

It's no surprise that the Popeye cartoons made spinach an icon for powerful health and strength.

If you are concerned about the health of your heart, spinach ranks high among the healthiest foods you can eat. It's packed with vitamin K, which contains a protein that keeps calcium from calcifying in your bloodstream, which offers you preventative measures against atherosclerosis, stroke, and cardiovascular disease. A cup of spinach gives you 100% of your daily requirement for this vitamin.

Spinach also contains peptides that are known to reduce high blood pressure. A cup of it has 20% of the fiber you need in a day and magnesium, which both promote healthy blood pressure. The antioxidant properties of vitamins A and C keep cholesterol from oxidizing, too.

TOMATOES

The tomato is one of those things for which the whole is better than the sum of its parts. Not only do they contain a lot of potent health benefits, but the combination of those elements work together to produce extra benefits. All four of the carotenoids, with their major anti-oxidant properties, are in tomatoes.

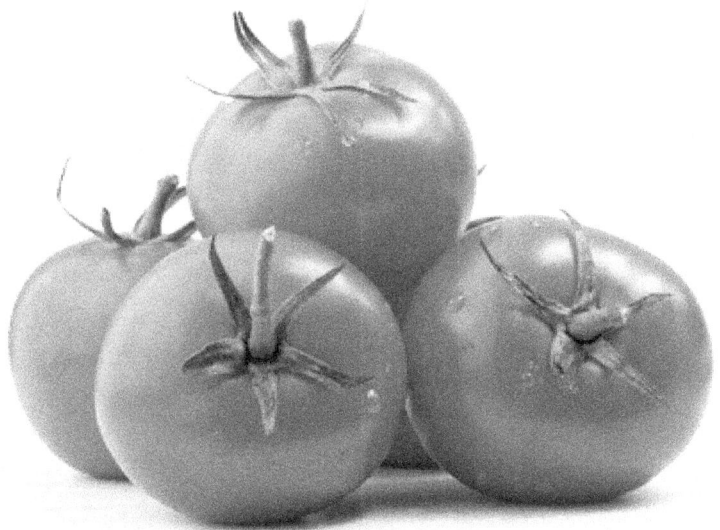

A study at Ohio State University found that when tomatoes are eaten together with healthy fats, "the body's absorption of the carotenoid phytochemicals in tomatoes can increase by two to 15 times." Tomatoes are also bursting with vitamins c and E, potassium, and flavonols.

The value of the Mediterranean diet is well known, and the tomato is a major ingredient in it. Researchers at the University of Athens recently reported that people who eat this diet show lower rates of fatal heart disease. The folates, niacin, and vitamin B6 in tomatoes are all valuable in lowering the risk of heart disease. Other studies have shown that eating 7 to 10 servings of tomatoes each week can lower the chances of getting heart disease by 29%, and that an 8 ounce glass of low-sodium tomato juice a day protects against thrombosis by keeping platelets from clotting. So if you have any heart problems, tomatoes offer one of the healthiest food choices you can make.

Sweet Potatoes

Sweet potatoes are a tasty and wonderfully beneficial addition to your diet, vegetables that have the sweetness of a dessert, but none of dessert's potential drawbacks.

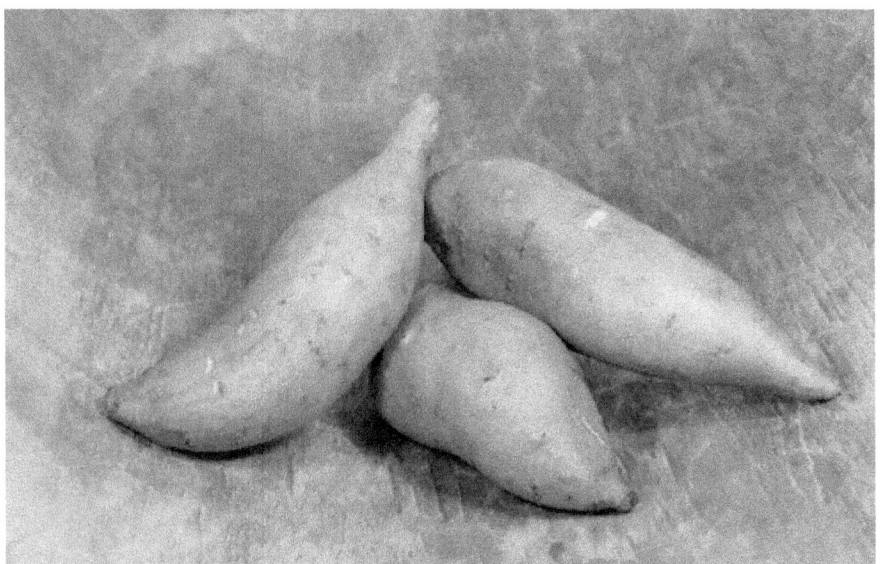

They offer a wealth of anti-oxidant carotenoids and phytonutrients that can cleanse the system of free radicals and heavy metals, a high concentration of vitamin A, and healthy doses of vitamin B6, vitamin C, and vitamin E. They also have a good amount of fiber, manganese, and potassium.

Inflammation, often the result of obesity, is directly related to the risk of heart disease. A team of researchers from the UK and Germany observed over 900 participants for 8 years and found that the livers of obese people in the study produced twice as much C-level proteins, and it is a direct correlation between high C-level protein counts and heart disease. A cup of cooked sweet potato contains enough vitamin C to lower risks of problems with your heart.

The rich vitamin B6 content prevents hardening of the arteries and keeps your blood vessels healthy and functioning smoothly. The potassium in sweet potatoes works to keep blood pressure down and flushes excess sodium out of your body. Potassium is also a potent electrolyte that keeps your heart beating in a natural rhythm. If the health of your heart is in question, you should definitely eat sweet potatoes often!

Red Peppers

The crunchy red bell pepper has a lot to offer you, besides the slightly sweet and mildly peppery fresh taste. Equally delicious raw or cooked, red bell peppers have few calories, virtually no fat, and a stellar offering of nutritious properties.

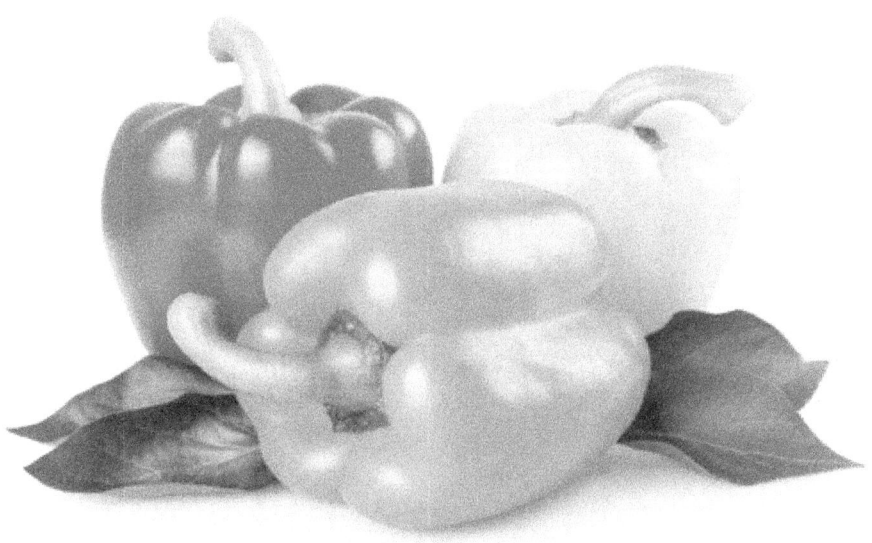

Capsaicin, the alkaloid compound also found in bell peppers' hotter relations, chili peppers, cuts down on bad cholesterol and triglycerides in your body, especially if you're struggling with weight issues.

A red pepper contains your entire daily vitamin C needs, and more vitamin A, that wonderful antioxidant, than required each day. Vitamin A is vital for synthesis of collagen, which keeps blood vessels and organs, including your heart, in good shape. Other vitamins found in red peppers include the B vitamins, E and K, and also fiber, folate, manganese, selenium, potassium, magnesium and carotene.

Louise Tremblay, a writer for Live Strong, wrote, "We expect to see antioxidant benefits specifically from bell peppers showing up in a wide variety of human health studies, including studies on prevention of cardiovascular disease." While they may be proved to have special benefit for your heart, in the future, there's no doubt that they are among the healthiest foods you can eat for maximizing your overall good health.

FIGS

The fig, a marvelous combination of
textures and sweetness, appears fresh in
markets in the late spring and provides a
taste treat into fall. When they're not
available seasonally, dried figs provide
the same powerful benefits to your body
all year long.

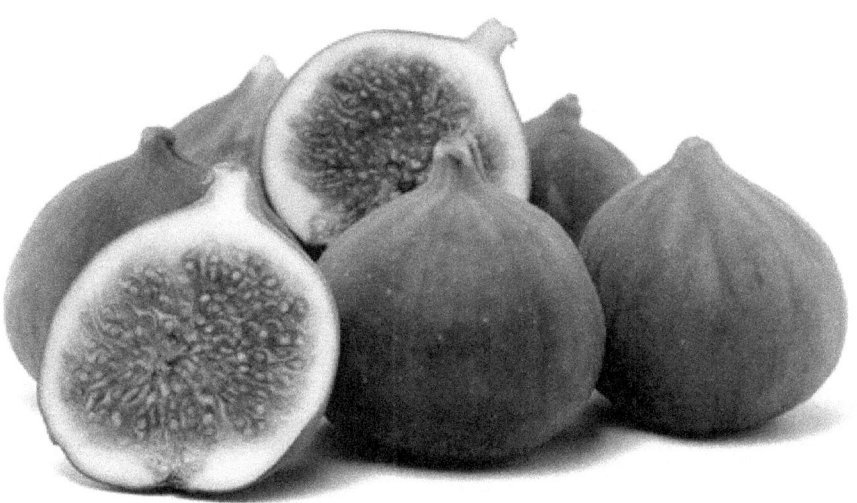

Figs are full of nutrients that promote
health, including potassium, fiber,
manganese, and vitamin B6, and they are
relatively low in calories. The same sized
serving of apples has half the iron
content; the same sized serving of

oranges has a quarter of the iron. The fig also delivers quite a bit of calcium.

The antioxidant power of figs is an advantage in any healthy diet and researchers believe that a diet rich in antioxidant foods promotes the health of your heart. Some researchers have determined that high fiber content, as you get in figs (especially the dark-skinned ones), is important for a diet designed to manage cardiovascular health, and it's also useful in helping you lose weight. The potassium in figs works to lower your blood pressure.

BLUEBERRIES

These tiny blue bundles of sweetness are a blessing if you like to snack. Low in calories and amazingly high in antioxidants, these berries actually offer so many benefits that you will want to have them around.

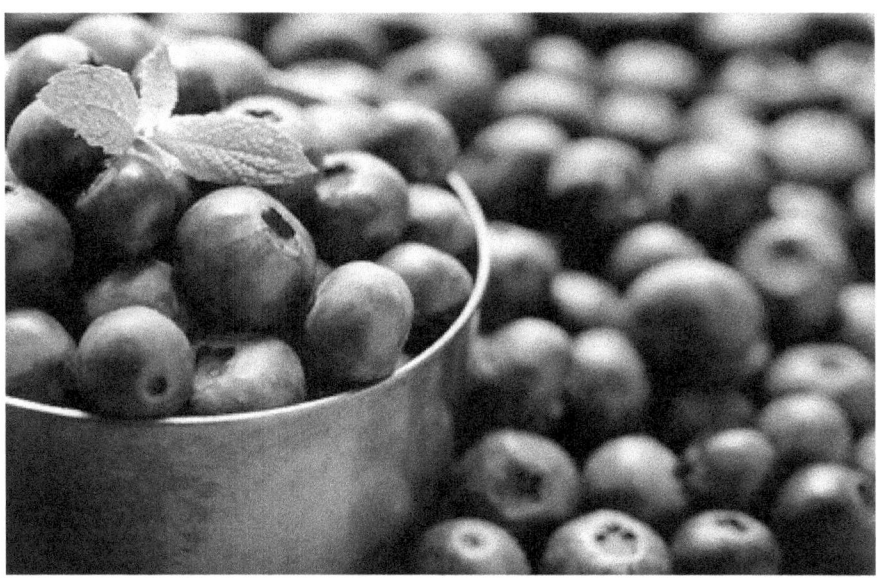

The World's Healthiest Foods site (http://www.whfoods.com) couldn't endorse them enough. They say that blueberries have "one of the highest antioxidant capacities among all fruits, vegetables, spices and seasonings."

Antioxidants, of course, keep free radicals from damaging the body, and they keep us young. But blueberries also have other properties that are equally important. One cup of blueberries contains almost 36% of the vitamin K we need each day, 25% of the manganese, 24% of the vitamin C, and over 14% of the fiber.

Amazingly, studies have recently shown that blueberries are one snack that you can eat plenty of and get a maximum of benefits in quantity. While you can get enough of certain nutrients in foods, you can never get enough antioxidants. Buying organically grown ones will provide even more advantages than commercially grown ones.

The antioxidant quality of blueberries boosts the health of your cardiovascular system in general, but blueberries give you even more support for the health of your heart. They've got an enzyme called eNOS that has been shown in recent clinical trials to improve the balance of the cardiovascular system. They also lower blood pressure. So eat them daily when they're in season. Researchers are recommending 3 cups a day.

APPLES

The health benefits of apples have been known for so long that their value has become part of conventional wisdom. Scientists have since identified the reasons why apple-eaters have always stayed so healthy.

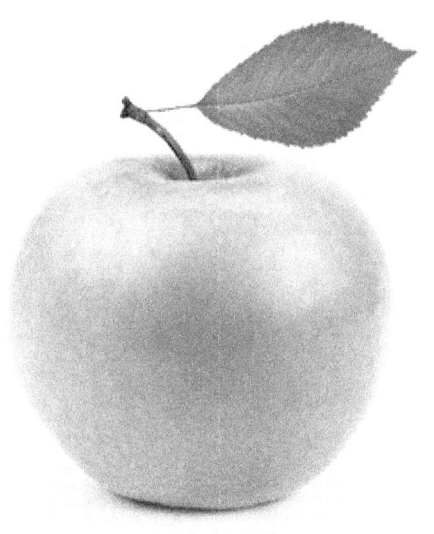

A recent study at Florida State University observed that women who ate a cup of apples every day for a year both lost weight and had lower cholesterol and risks for heart disease.

The FSU researchers think that the antioxidants and pectin in apples are responsible for the improved health markers. An apple also contains 30% of the fiber you need in a day, as well as phytonutrients and polyphenols. Each color of apple contains different types and strength of these vital nutrients, and the benefits are mostly in the skin. A medium apple has no fat, no cholesterol, and only about 50 calories. Eating all the different colors provides a full range of their nutritional value.

Kerri-Ann Jennings, the nutrition editor at Eating Well Magazine, wrote, "the Iowa Women's Health Study reported that, among the 34,000-plus women it's been tracking for nearly 20 years, apples were associated with a lower risk of death from both coronary heart disease and cardiovascular disease." Another study done in Finland found that regularly eating apples reduces the risk of stroke.

Dark Chocolate

It's a great surprise when something we think is bad for us turns out to be very good. Dark chocolate is one of those great surprises. Rich in antioxidant flavonols, dark chocolate provides the same benefits found in antioxidant fruits and vegetables, but it is best eaten in much smaller amounts.

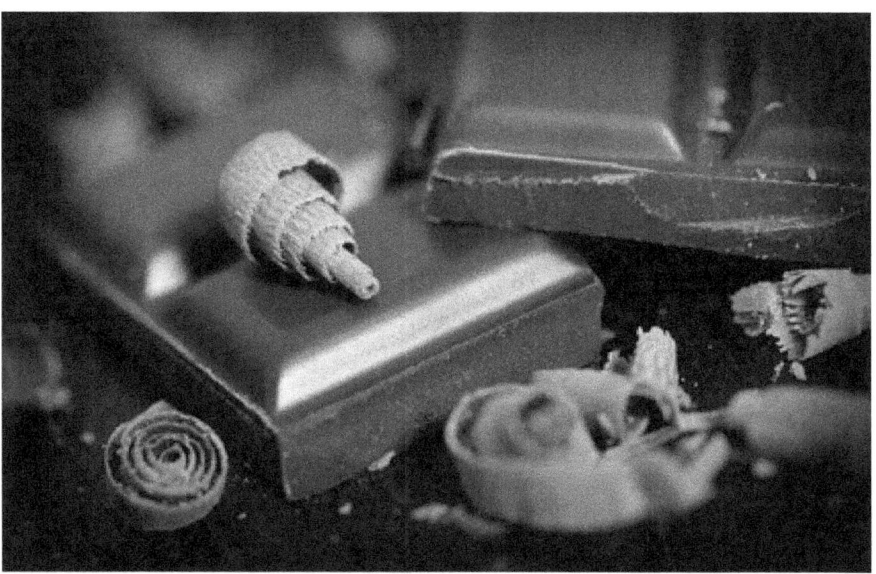

Dr, Mee Young Hong of San Diego State University recently reported findings from a study on the effects of eating dark chocolate on your health. Participants ate 1.7 ounces daily of either dark or white chocolate. Those eating dark chocolate showed a 20% improvement of bad cholesterol and a 20% improvement of good cholesterol after only 15 days. Nutritional epidemiologist Dr. Eric Ding, an instructor at Harvard Medical School, adds that other studies of have shown that it also lowers blood pressure.

Evidence is growing that dark chocolate improves your cardiovascular health. The value of antioxidants is clear, but research is showing that the flavonal content, besides lowering blood pressure, makes blood flow better to the heart, improves the blood's ability to clot, and reduces the stickiness of blood platelets.

ASIAN PEARS

The Asian pear is sometimes mistaken for a related, but different fruit called the pear apple, because unlike most of the familiar pear varieties usually seen in supermarkets, it's actually shaped more like an apple.

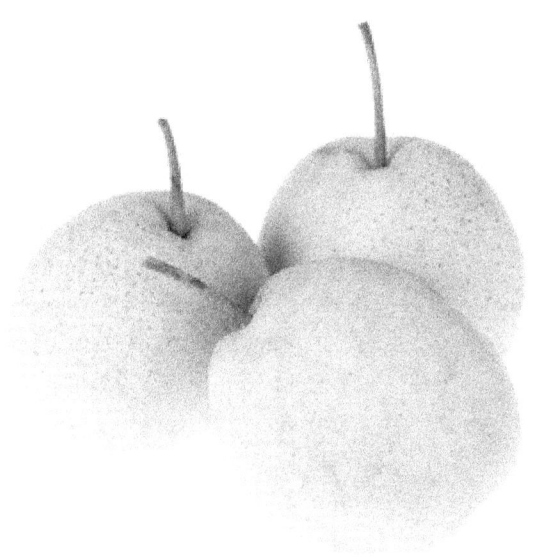

Unlike softer varieties of pears, the Asian pear has a crunchier consistency and a thicker skin. But you should eat that skin - recent research has found that the skin is where the most phenolic phytonutrients are, as many as 3 or 4

times as much as in the sweet inside of the fruit.

One Asian pear is low in calories, averaging about 50 calories in a medium-sized fruit. It contains about four-fifths of all the vitamin C you need in a day, 14% of the vitamin K and 22% of the fiber. They're rich in flavonols and carotenoids, and are considered to be hypoallergenic.

All pears have qualities that support a healthy heart, although not in the same ways we tend to think of, like having strong antioxidant or anti-inflammatory properties. They decrease cholesterol synthesis because of the way their particular fibers combine with bile acids, and of all the fruits, only pineapples and bananas topped pears in this capacity. They lower blood cholesterol, and the high fiber content creates a sensation of fullness, a benefit for weight loss and overall health.

LYCHEE

The name lychee means "gift for a joyful life" in Chinese. Somehow, even without the benefits of modern biochemistry to inform them, the Chinese ancients knew that eating lychee would make them feel good - and they were right.

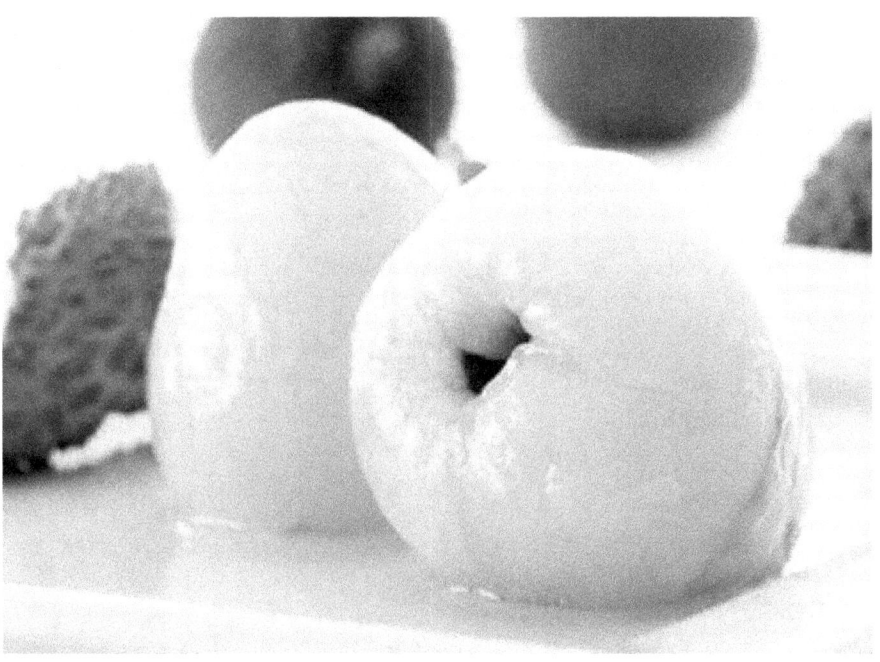

Lychees, often called lychee or litchi nuts, are actually berries, even though they are contained in a thin, external shell of a red or pink hue. They combine a heady perfume and sweet, clean taste that hints at the powerful combination of nutrients they contain. They're extremely high in vitamin C. A cup of lychees has more than the minimum of your daily requirement of C, and researchers in China now say that it has more antioxidant strength than the vitamin itself. Other beneficial elements in lychees are folate, niacin, vitamin B-6, thiamin, and riboflavin.

Lychees are very high in potassium content, and potassium is important in maintaining low blood pressure and a healthy level of water in your system. The antioxidant boost in these super fruits also offers benefits for your overall health, notably the functioning of your heart.

Guava

The guava is a fruit that's not seen in most market fruit displays, but it really ought to be, as this fruit packs more nutrients than most. With zero cholesterol, very little fat content, and few calories, a guava provides almost 400% of all the vitamin C you need daily, and more lycopene than tomatoes.

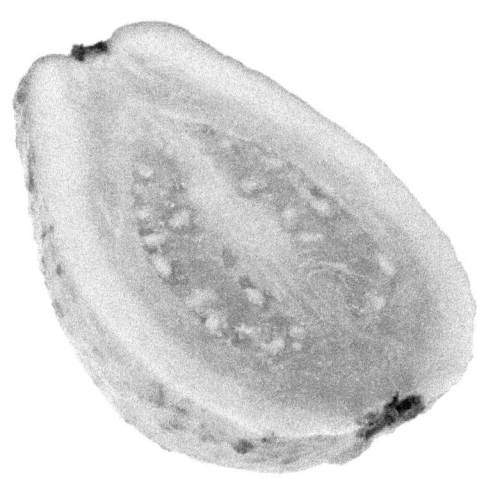

If that weren't impressive enough, it also gives you 14% of your daily fiber, 12.5% of your folates, and significant amounts of vitamin A, pantothenic acids, carotenes, and potassium. Smaller amounts of calcium and magnesium, copper, manganese, phosphorus, zinc, and selenium are also found in this nutritious small fruit.

Anything with as many antioxidants as the guava is certainly beneficial for your heart. The fiber content helps to keep cholesterol in check, and the high potassium to low sodium ratio of its properties helps keep your blood pressure down. The Linus Pauling Institute says that diets high in vitamin C are a preventative against heart disease - and guavas have an extraordinary amount of it.

TOFU AND EDAMAME

Tofu and Edamame is an excellent source of plant-based protein. A half-cup serving of firm tofu is 10.7% protein, and contains only 5% fat. "Silken" tofu, which is not as firm, is 5.3% protein, and only 2% fat.

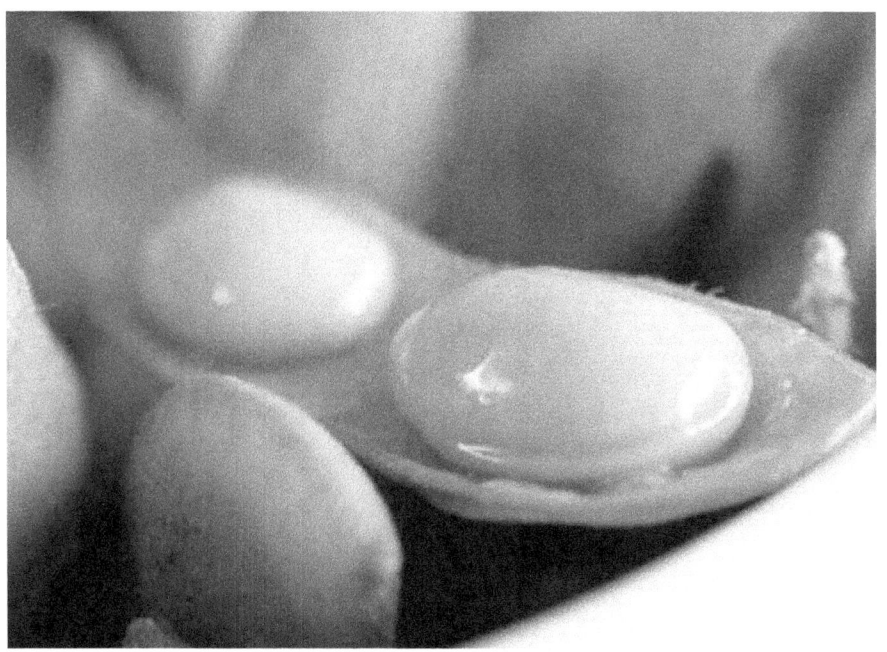

A recent study at the University of Hong Kong showed that like other plant-based proteins, it lowers levels of "bad" cholesterol. The high level of isoflavones in tofu may be associated with a lower risk of heart disease. It is also high in calcium content.

Tofu is made from mature soybeans, but edamame are the immature green beans that have been boiled. They are high in fiber and lower in fat than a comparable serving of firm tofu, but the fat content is monounsaturated or polyunsaturated, and contains a small percentage of omega-3 fatty acids. A half-cup of these beans gives you 10% of the vitamin C, 10% of the iron, 8% of the vitamin A, and 4% of the calcium you need in a day.

2.2 DASH

Here is a little more from "Your Guide to Lowering Blood Pressure with DASH":

What you eat affects your chances of developing high blood pressure (hypertension). Research shows that high blood pressure can be prevented - and lowered - by following the Dietary Approaches to Stop Hypertension (DASH) eating plan, which includes eating less salt and sodium.

The DASH eating plan is rich in fruits, vegetables, fat-free or low-fat milk and milk products, whole grains, fish, poultry, beans, seeds, and nuts. It also contains less salt and sodium; sweets, added sugars, and sugar-containing beverages; fats; and red meats than the typical American diet. This heart healthy way of eating is also lower in saturated fat, trans-fat, and cholesterol and rich in nutrients that are associated with lowering blood pressure - mainly potassium, magnesium, and calcium, protein, and fiber.

How do I make the DASH

The DASH eating plan requires no special foods and has no hard-to-follow recipes. It simply calls for a certain number of daily servings from various food groups.

The number of servings depends on the number of calories you're allowed each day. Your calorie level depends on your age and, especially, how active you are. Think of this as an energy balance system - if you want to maintain your current weight, you should take in only as many calories as you burn by being physically active. If you need to lose weight, eat fewer calories than you burn or increase your activity level to burn more calories than you eat.

3. PHYSICAL ACTIVITY

"Your Guide to Lowering Blood Pressure with DASH" also has a few things to say about physical activity:

Being physically active is one of the most important things you can do to prevent or control high blood pressure. It also helps to reduce your risk of heart disease. It doesn't take a lot of effort to become physically active. All you need is 30 minutes of moderate-level physical activity on most days of the week. Examples of such activities are brisk walking, bicycling, raking leaves, and gardening.

You can even divide the 30 minutes into shorter periods of at least 10 minutes each.

For instance: Use stairs instead of an elevator, get off a bus one or two stops early, or park your car at the far end of the lot at work. If you already engage in 30 minutes of moderate-level physical activity a day, you can get added benefits by doing more. Engage in a moderate-level activity for a longer period each day or engage in a more vigorous activity.

Most people don't need to see a doctor before they start a moderate-level physical activity. You should check first with your doctor if you have heart trouble or have had a heart attack, if you're over age 50 and are not used to moderate-level physical activity, if you have a family history of heart disease at an early age, or if you have any other serious health problem.

3.1 EVERYDAY

There are plenty of opportunities for some physical activity in your everyday life. I started to take a different look at some activities I used to consider as very boring, and turned them into a part of my exercise program. Some examples:

CLEANING

I started looking at cleaning as a form of exercise. I did one 30-60 minutes vacuuming and cleaning session each week.

DO THE LAWN

Like the cleaning, I looked at this as a good exercise. It took 60-90 minutes, in a slope – very good work-out. In the summer this is a once-a-week activity.

EVENING WALK

Instead of eating a big evening meal, I went for walks in my neighborhood.

3.2 WORKOUTS

I felt I needed more activity than my everyday routines could offer, so I designed a set of workouts to choose from. Depending on my mood or the weather I alternate between indoor and outdoor activity.

I also like to do different things, so I needed some variety. It was important for me that these exercises was

- Easy accessible exercises – limited time spent before and after the actual workouts
- Affordable – no expensive gyms or gear.

Whatever I do – I like to measure my performance and progress – and this made it easier to see if my plan was working along the way.

These are the workouts I do:

JOGGING

Jogging has been around as a form of exercise for a long time. No wonder - all you need is a good pair of shoes. Many think jogging is a bit boring – running around thinking of how long it will take to finish.

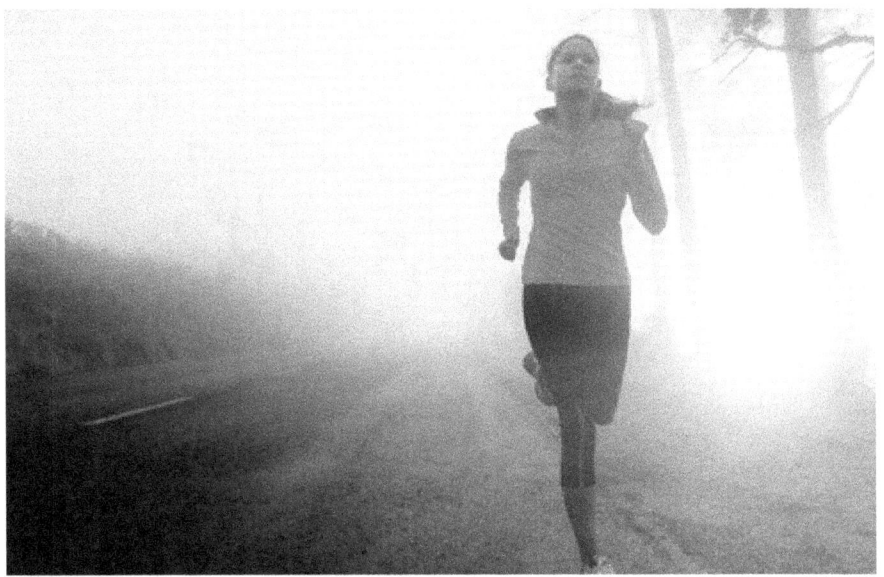

But you can make this a bit more interesting by varying the long trips with some interval training.

You need not be a top athlete to benefit from interval training.

The point is that you should challenge your capacity and compete with yourself.

It's like quality work in your business – focus on continuous improvement.

1. *Long distance* - Maybe the most common way to go jogging. You go along at a fixed pace. The heart rate should be at 50-60% of max. For variation I use 5-6 tracks of different lengths.

2. *Intervals* - The most intense parts of the interval training should be 70-80% of max. I normally use intervals of 4x4 minutes.

I often do 4 minutes walking - 4 minutes running. Repeating intervals for 30 minutes or more.

3. *Short intervals* - Lately there has been much focus on the effects of intense exercise in short intervals, such as these

- 30 seconds max - 90 sec rest
- 20 sec max - 40 sec rest
- 40 sec max - 20 sec rest

Sometimes I do a very simple interval routine:

- Run 100 yards/meters close to max, slightly uphill. Walk back and repeat 10-15 times or more if you like.

UPHILL WALKING

There are few things that challenge your body more than the uphills. If you prefer walking to other activities, but still want to make it a form of training - and more than just easy exercise - this program could be for you. This is good for the heart, lungs, legs, back and abdominals.

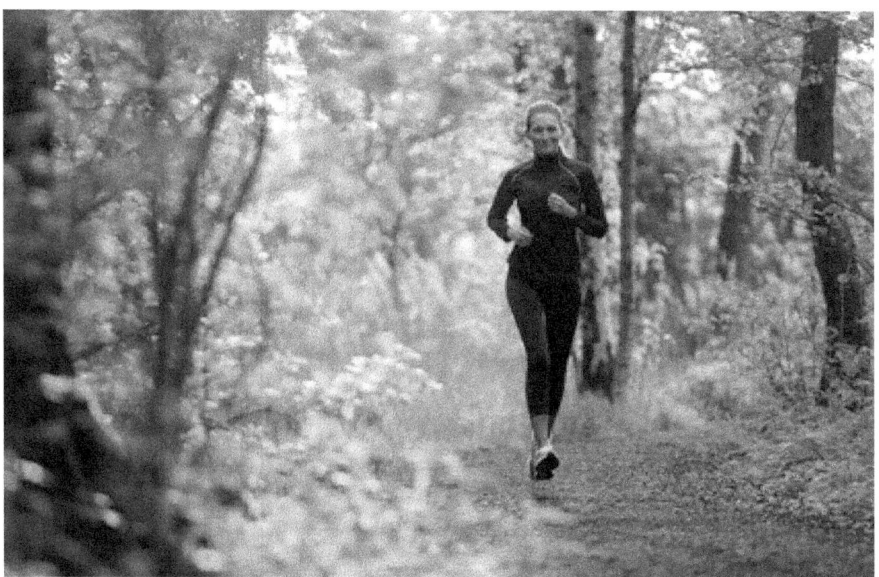

Duration up to 30 min (not including the trip back). Find an uphill - preferably of a certain length and gradient. Set goals for how long you will use to the top or how far to go in a given time. The point is that you should measure your progress over time. Your heart rate should be pretty high - 70-80 percent of max. I vary between different trips, like these:

Do the walk in one sequence.

Find a hill you may eventually walk continuously for up to 30 minutes.

Do intervals.

If it is a long uphill with continuous gradient, break up the trip in regular intervals, and slow down in between. I walk different slopes with varying gradients, so I let the slope decide my intervals.

Walk in the terrain

I think it's good training to walk outside the forest roads and trails, into more rugged terrain. I recommend good hiking boots when you do this.

STATIONARY BIKE

During winter this is my most valued exercise equipment. I have it in my living room, so it's very easy jump on it for a short workout.

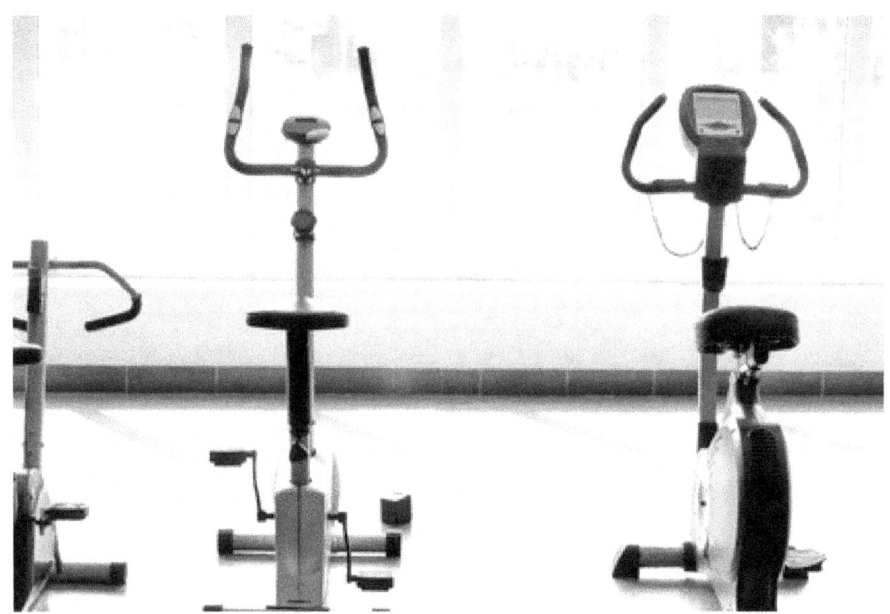

I use it when I watch the news – morning or evening – and often as a warm up for my kettlebells workout. To make it a bit more "interesting" I put in a lot of variations in these workouts.

The routines I apply on the bike are very much the same as on my jogging routines:

- long distance
- interval
- short/intense interval.

I also vary the resistance and the duration of the workouts.

I normally do the bike 2-3 times a week.

KETTLEBELLS

This is my new favorite workout. I bought "Kettlebells for Dummies" – as they claimed these tempting benefits:

- Work all your muscle groups at once
- Improve your strength, endurance, flexibility, agility, and body alignment
- Burn fat, build lean muscle, and achieve core strength

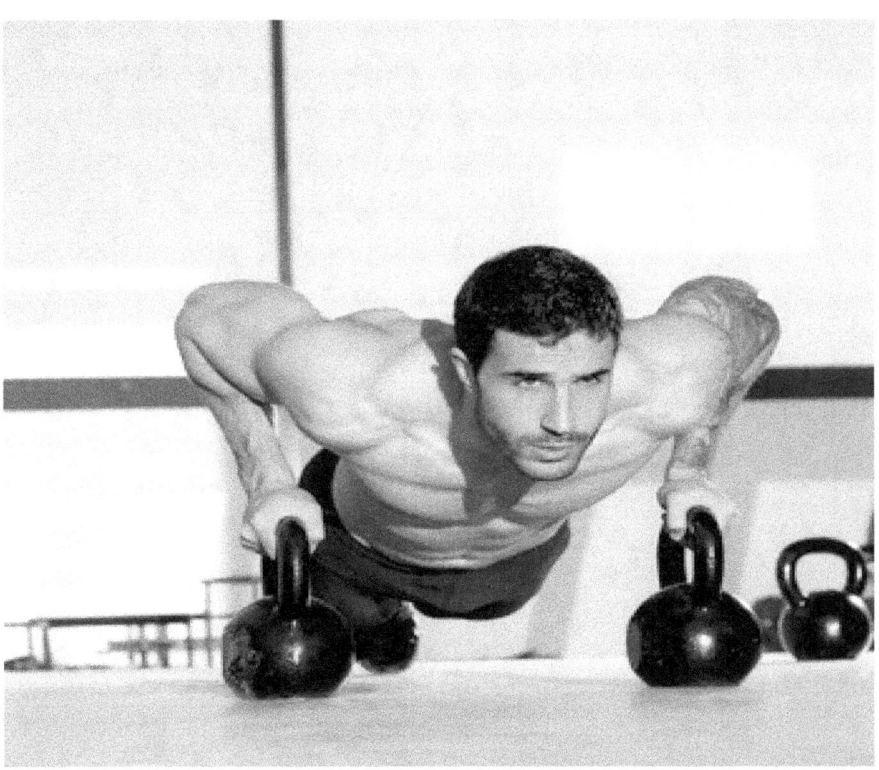

In addition they promised to boost my metabolism and lose weight, which was one of my primary objectives.

But I'm very satisfied with this simple and affordable little piece of iron. I have been using different kinds of exercise equipment for many years – this one is the most effective tool I have ever come across.

There's a range of different exercises you can do. I have a couple of programs with 8-10 exercises I try to do 2-3 times a week. Each workout is from 20 to 40 minutes.

If you are new to Kettlebells, I strongly recommend you to get some basic instructions on how to use them before you start your workouts. I did not, and got a back injury that took a few weeks to heal.

FLOWIN

A friend of mine suggested this one. I've used this as an alternative to kettlebells sometimes. And believe me – it works! If you want to get quick results from your training, without going outside your door, then you should test FLOWIN.

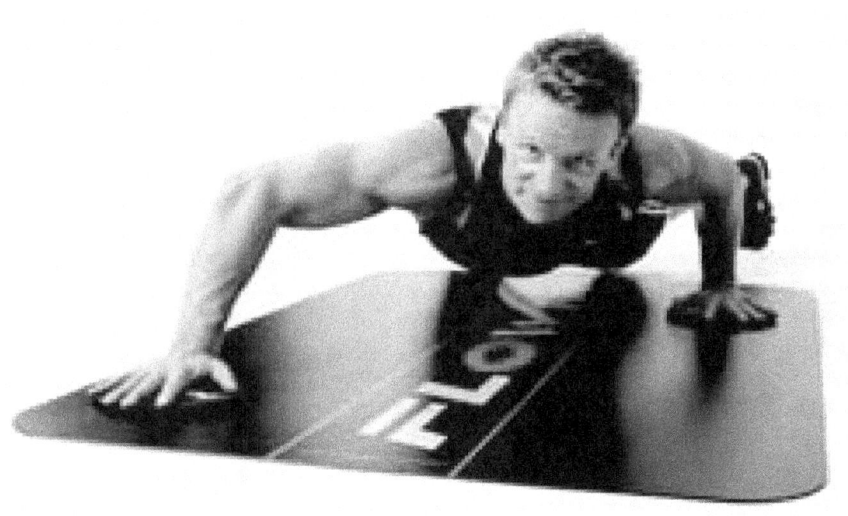

A specially designed flowin plate and five so-called pads - is all it takes for you to get started. Less than half an hour is required to give your muscles a good workout. Without lifting a single weight. With FLOWIN the resistance is your body weight, combined with the friction created between the pads and the plate.

By means of pads, which are shaped differently for the different body parts, you create a movement on the plate. With hands, feet and knees on the pillows you create support points that are moved on and off the plate. The exercises are actually similar to normal strength and stability exercises, and have much in common with Pilates and conventional core muscle training.

The big difference is that, thanks to the base, you can work more with your movements and create dynamic exercises instead of static work. This form of exercise is also well suited to train endurance and stamina.

3.3 HOW TO GO 30MAD

There seems to be consensus today among the different authorities on health and exercise. From what I read I understand that:

- The minimum amount of exercise per day should be 30 minutes.
- 30 minutes a day is enough to give you good, and long lasting health effects
- Exercising more than this only gives marginally better results
- A lot of everyday activities can be counted as exercise.

So I started to think of 30 minutes activities as 30MAD. Anyone can invest 30 minutes a day in their own health.

How to go about 30MAD?

Some examples of very simple 30MAD activities are:

1. Walking

Walking slowly around the house might not be a killer activity, but many of us actually have to go to work, to the shop or some other place. For some of us it could mean walking instead of taking the car. Or you could jump off the bus or the train a little earlier on your way to work - or back home.

If this is not suitable, go for a walk around your neighborhood in the evening, or take a walk in the nearby forest.

2. Bicycle

For many people, this is their everyday transportation, and something to consider for many of us. So easy to take a detour just to get these 30MAD!

3. Home activities

There are lot of activities in your home that can be counted as exercise - like washing, vacuuming, redecorating and gardening. The effect of these activities (like all others) obviously depends on the intensity applied!

But there are numerous ways to do some 30MAD activity. Check my list for ideas. The list shows 30 different activities, enough to choose from for most of us.

30 MAD LIST

1. Bicycle
2. Bosu
3. Car wash
4. Chopping wood
5. Cleaning
6. Exercise bands
7. Flowin
8. Gardening
9. Gliding discs
10. Gym
11. Home Gym 2000
12. House redecoration
13. House rehabilitation
14. Jogging
15. Jump ropes
16. Kettlebells
17. Mowing the lawn
18. Punching bag
19. Rock ring)
20. Ropes(trx)
21. Rowing
22. Running
23. Skiing
24. Snow Shoes
25. Stability ball
26. Stationary Bike
27. Swimming
28. Uphill walking
29. Walking
30. Walk the dog

4. EQUIPMENT

There is a lot of equipment and gear you can use for your physical activity. I will give some tips on the equipment I have used.

The point here is that it's affordable, but don't make it too affordable!

My point is – as an example - that a pair of running shoes should be of good quality, so I don't go for the cheapest ones, for two reasons:

- I want to have good protection from injuries

- Quality last longer – so in the long run this is good economy

4.1 RUNNING SHOES

As with all footwear, choose good quality. Avoid buying the cheapest shoes. Walking, jogging or running - it is important that the shoes fit your foot, have proper cushioning, support and are appropriate to the circumstances you intend to use them.

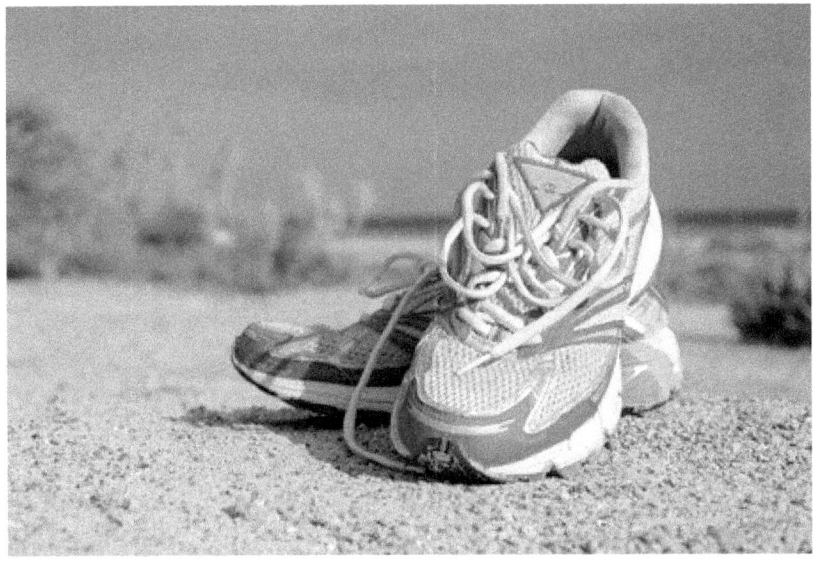

Are they for use in the sunny, dry summer on asphalt - or will you use them in the forest on cold and rainy autumn evenings. When choosing shoes, think of how you will use them.

Whatever the use, it is important also to think about your weight. Be sure to have a cushioning which is calibrated for your weight. If you are thinking of using the shoes in any weather and most of the year, consider shoes with Gore Tex. It is important to stay dry on your feet as long as possible. As long as your feet are dry and not least comfortable, it's a lot easier to take a trip - even in wet or bad weather.

4.2 KETTLEBELLS

They come in different designs, sizes and weights. And of course prices.

I prefer the one-piece iron, with a handle wide enough to put both hands into if needed.

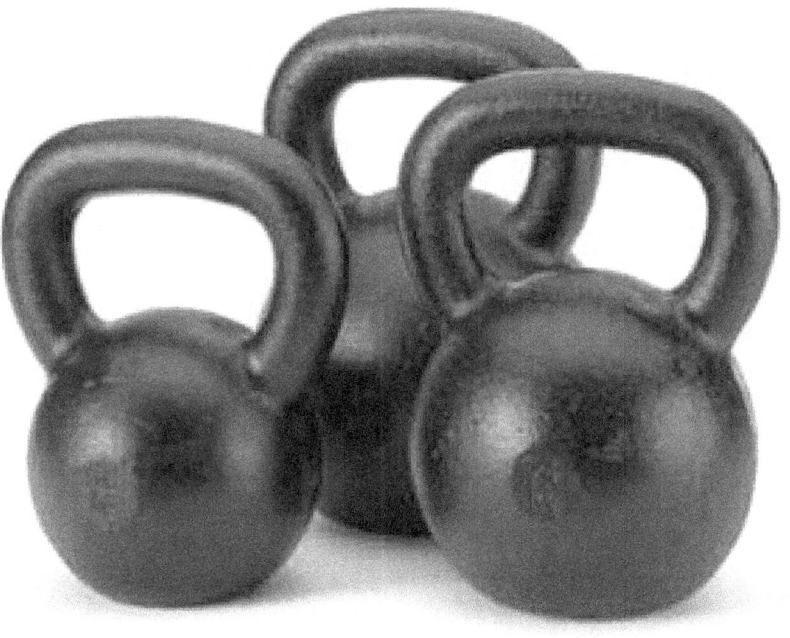

As a start you only need one. And don't start too heavy. Get some instructions and test the kettlebell before you decide

on the weight. If you like this kind of
workouts you can expand your range of
kettlebells later.

4.3 STATIONARY BIKE

Many look at this as a little boring piece of equipment. You sit there for as you don't know how long, and nothing really happens except you get even more bored. But I have come to think of this little work horse in more positive ways.

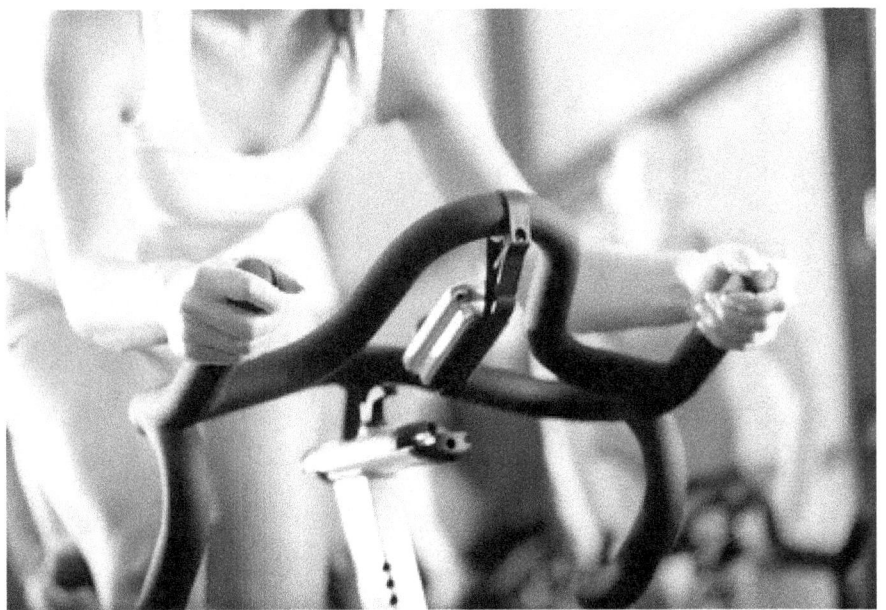

Why use a stationary bike?

It's very easy to use it. It often comes with a timer and a heart rate monitor, so it's easy to see if you keep your intensity at the right level. If you put it in an easily accessible - and visible place - in your house, chances are that you will use it more. It's also very easy to vary your routine here. Instead of just going at the same pace for the whole session you can implement your own intervals of different resistance, speed and duration. Many bikes also have different programs you can use.

4.4 FLOWIN

If you want to get quick results from your training, without going outside your door, then try FLOWIN - a Swedish training concept based on efficient and functional workout for exercisers and athletes of all levels.

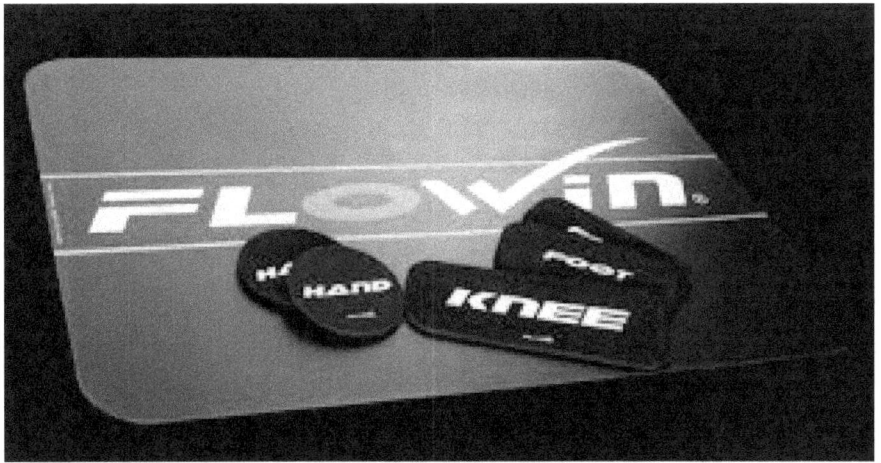

The equipment is a plate and five so-called pads. By means of the pads, which are shaped differently for the different body parts, you create a movement on the plate. With hands, feet and knees on the pillows you create support points that are moved on and off the plate.

This form of exercise is well suited to train core muscles, strength, stability, endurance and stamina.

When working with your own body weight as the load, it's up to you how heavy your workout becomes. Factors that determine this includes how much pressure you put on the pads, how much support you have, how far you go in the various exercises, how many repetitions you perform and at what speed. As long as you are using your own body weight the risk of injury is very low.

Using FLOWIN you don't exercise each individual muscle. Instead, the focus is, as with other functional training, to activate many muscle groups at once and let them interact with each other. You work with your body the way it works in everyday life or on the sports field.

5. FACTS

According to World Health Organization and U. S. Department of Health and Human Services, high blood pressure, which is blood pressure higher than 140/90 mmHg, affects more than one in three adults worldwide. It is considered directly responsible for almost 13% of all global deaths. Almost as many have prehypertension, which is blood pressure between 120/80 and 140/89 mmHg. This increases their chances of developing high blood pressure and its complications.

High blood pressure is dangerous because it makes your heart work too hard, hardens the walls of your arteries and can cause the brain to hemorrhage or the kidneys to function poorly or not function at all. If not controlled, high blood pressure can lead to heart and kidney disease, stroke and blindness.

I have sampled a few fact sheets from "Your Guide to Lowering Blood Pressure" (U.S: Department of Health and Human Services):

5.1 RISK FACTORS

High blood pressure is one of several risk
factors for developing a heart disease

RISK FACTORS FOR HEART DISEASE

Risk factors are conditions or behaviors that increase your chances of developing a disease. When you have more than one risk factor for heart disease, your risk of developing heart disease greatly multiplies. So if you have high blood pressure, you need to take action. Fortunately, you can control most heart disease risk factors.

RISK FACTORS YOU CAN CONTROL:
- High blood pressure
- Abnormal cholesterol
- Tobacco use
- Diabetes
- Overweight
- Physical inactivity

RISK FACTORS BEYOND YOUR CONTROL:
- Age (55 or older for men; 65 or older for women)
- Family history of early heart disease (having a father or brother diagnosed with heart disease before age 55 or having a mother or sister diagnosed before age 65)

5.2 BLOOD PRESSURE LEVELS

CATEGORY	SYSTOLIC† (MMHG)‡		DIASTOLIC† (MMHG)‡	RESULT
Normal	less than 120	and	less than 80	Good for you!
Prehypertension	120–139	or	80–89	Your blood pressure could be a problem. Make changes in what you eat and drink, be physically active, and lose extra weight. If you also have diabetes, see your doctor.
Hypertension	140 or higher	or	90 or higher	You have high blood pressure. Ask your doctor or nurse how to control it.

* For adults ages 18 and older who are not on medicine for high blood pressure and do not have a short-term serious illness. *Source: The Seventh Report of the Joint National Committee on Prevention, Detection, Evaluation, and Treatment of High Blood Pressure;* NIH Publication No. 03-5230, National High Blood Pressure Education Program, May 2003.
† If systolic and diastolic pressures fall into different categories, overall status is the higher category.
‡ Millimeters of mercury

A blood pressure level of 140/90 mmHg or higher is considered high. About two-thirds of people over age 65 have high blood pressure. If your blood pressure is between 120/80 mmHg and 139/89 mmHg, then you have prehypertension. This means that you don't have high blood pressure now but are likely to develop it in the future unless you adopt the healthy lifestyle changes.

People who do not have high blood pressure at age 55 face a 90 percent chance of developing it during their lifetimes. So high blood pressure is a condition that most people will have at some point in their lives.

Both numbers in a blood pressure test are important, but for people who are age 50 or older, systolic pressure gives the most accurate diagnosis of high blood pressure. Systolic pressure is the top number in a blood pressure reading. It is high if it is 140 mmHg or above.

5.3 BMI

Take a look at this chart and see if you can find your BMI. Three years ago I was outside – to the right!!

BODY MASS INDEX

Here is a chart for men and women that gives BMI for various heights and weights.* To use the chart, find your height in the left-hand column labeled Height. Move across to your body weight. The number at the top of the column is the BMI for your height and weight.

BMI	21	22	23	24	25	26	27	28	29	30	31
HEIGHT (FEET AND INCHES)					BODY WEIGHT (POUNDS)						
4' 10"	100	105	110	115	119	124	129	134	138	143	148
5' 0"	107	112	118	123	128	133	138	143	148	153	158
5' 2"	115	120	126	131	136	142	147	153	158	164	169
5' 4"	122	128	134	140	145	151	157	163	169	174	180
5' 6"	130	136	142	148	155	161	167	173	179	186	192
5' 8"	138	144	151	158	164	171	177	184	190	197	203
5' 10"	146	153	160	167	174	181	188	195	202	209	216
6' 0"	154	162	169	177	184	191	199	206	213	221	228
6' 2"	163	171	179	186	194	202	210	218	225	233	241
6' 4"	172	180	189	197	205	213	221	230	238	246	254

* Weight is measured with underwear but no shoes.

WHAT DOES YOUR BMI MEAN?

CATEGORY	BMI	RESULT
Normal weight	18.5–24.9	Good for you! Try not to gain weight.
Overweight	25–29.9	Do not gain any weight, especially if your waist measurement is high. You need to lose weight if you have two or more risk factors for heart disease. (See box 1.)
Obese	30 or greater	You need to lose weight. Lose weight slowly — about 1/2 pound to 2 pounds a week. See your doctor or a registered dietitian if you need help.

Source: Clinical Guidelines on the Identification, Evaluation, and Treatment of Overweight and Obesity in Adults: The Evidence Report; NIH Publication No. 98-4083, National Heart, Lung, and Blood Institute, in cooperation with the National Institute of Diabetes and Digestive and Kidney Diseases, National Institutes of Health, June 1998.

References

1) World Health Organization

http://www.who.int/gho/ncd/risk_factors/blood_pressure_prevalence/en/

2) U. S. Department of Health and Human Services, National Institute of Health, National Heart, Lung and Blood Institute.

- NIH Publication No. 03-5232.
- NIH Publication No. 06-5834.

http://www.nhlbi.nih.gov/health/public/heart/hbp/dash/index.htm

3) Food references

- Alvizouri-Munoz, M., Carranza-Madrigal, J., Herrera-Abarca, F. Amezcua-Gastelum, H. (1992). Effects of avocado as a source of monounsaturated fatty acids on plasma lipid levels. Arch Med Res. 1992 Winter: 23(4), pp. 163-7.
- Center For Disease Control. Polyunsaturated Fats and Monounsaturated Fats. http://www.cdc.gov/nutrition/everyone/basics/fat/unsaturatedfat.html
- Coulson, A.M. (1999) Dietary fatty acids in plant based diets. Am J Clin Nutr 1999;70(suppl):512S–5S.
- Saturated Fat. Center for Disease Control: http://www.cdc.gov/nutrition/everyone/basics/fat/saturatedfat.html
- Lichtenstein, A. H. et al. (2006). AHA Scientific Statement Diet and Lifestyle Recommendations Revision 2006. Circulation. 2006;114:82-96.

111

- Sifferlin, A. (2012). Skim Milk Drinkers Rejoice: You May Have a Lower Stroke Risk! Time (online). http://healthland.time.com/2012/04/20/skim-milk-drinkers-rejoice-you-may-have-a-lower-stroke-risk/
- Mozaffarian, D,, Eric B. Rimm, E. (2006). Fish Intake, Contaminants, and Human Health: Evaluating the Risks and the Benefits. JAMA. 2006;296(15):1885-1899.
- Kris-Etherton, P.M., Harris, W.S., Appel, L.J. ((2003). Omega-3 Fatty Acids and Cardiovascular Disease: New Recommendations From the American Heart Association. Arterioscler Thromb Vasc Biol. 2003;23:151-152.
- Rehmeyer, J. (2007). Salmon Safety. Science News, January 15, 2007. www.sciencenews.org/view/generic/id/8133/.../Salmon_Safety
- Celentano, J. C. (2009). Where Do Eggs Fit in a Heart-healthy Diet? Am J Lifestyle Med. 2009;3(4):274-278.
- Oz, M. (2011) The Oz Diet. Time Magazine, September 12, 2011. Healthy Ways to Help Achieve New Year's Goals in January and Throughout the Year
- Source: Obesity, Fitness & Wellness Week. (Jan. 7, 2012): p331.
- Pressner, A. 10 Surprising Health Benefits of Yogurt, Prevention. http://www.fitnessmagazine.com/recipes/healthy-eating/nutrition/health-benefits-of-yogurt/
- McIntosh, G., Roupas, P., Roule P.(2006). Cheese, omega-3 fatty acids, conjugated linoleic acid and human health. Australian Journal of Dairy Technology, vol. 61, no. 2.
- Kabagambe, E. K., Bavlin, A., Ruis-Navarez, E., Siles, X., Campos, H. (2005). Decreased Consumption of Dried Mature Beans Is Positively Associated with Urbanization and Nonfatal Acute Myocardial Infarction. J. Nutr. July 1, 2005, vol. 135 no. 7, pp. 1770-1775.
- French, R. (2011) Nutritional Facts for dried beans. Livestrong. http://www.livestrong.com/article/296071-nutritional-facts-for-dried-beans/.

- Daniel, C.R., Cross, A. J., Keobnick, C.,Sinha, R. (2011). Trends in red meat consumption in the United States. Public Health Nutr. Vol 14, No.4. pp. 575-583.
- Grogan, M. Grass-fed beef: What are the heart-health benefits? http://www.mayoclinic.com/health/grass-fed-beef/AN02053
- Mayo Clinic. Cuts of beef: A guide to the leanest selections. http://www.mayoclinic.com/health/cuts-of-beef/MY01387
- Garlic: http://www.webmd.com/vitamins-supplements/ingredientmono-300-GARLIC.aspx?activeIngredientId=300&activeIngredientName=GARLIC
- Garlic Nutrition Facts: http://www.nutrition-and-you.com/garlic.html
- Bender, R. G. (2012). Why You Should Go Nuts for Nuts. Everydayhealth.com http://www.everydayhealth.com/diet-and-nutrition/0406/why-you-should-go-nuts-for-nuts.aspx#.
- Ros, E. (2009).Nuts and novel biomarkers of cardiovascular disease. Am J Clin Nutr, 2009;89(suppl):1649S–56S.
- Stein, N. (2011). Roasted Nuts & High Blood Pressure. http://www.livestrong.com/article/464800-roasted-nuts-high-blood-pressure/?utm_source=popslideshow&utm_medium=a1
- Griffin, R. M. (2012). The New Low-Cholesterol Diet: Oatmeal & Oat Bran. http://www.webmd.com/cholesterol-management/features/the-new-cholesterol-diet-oatmeal-oat-bran
- Handler, J. (2012). Oatmeal Nutrition Facts. http://www.mnn.com/food/healthy-eating/stories/oatmeal-nutrition-facts
- Mcgee, E. The Benefits of Flaxseed. http://www.webmd.com/diet/features/benefits-of-flaxseed
- Foster, S. Flaxseed and Flaxseed Oil. National Center for Complementary and Alternative Medicine. http://nccam.nih.gov/health/flaxseed/ataglance.htm

- Sheehan, K. (2011). Should You Drink a Shot of Olive Oil a Day? http://www.livestrong.com/article/508869-should-you-drink-a-shot-of-olive-oil-a-day/
- Olive Oil Nutrition Facts. http://www.nutrition-and-you.com/olive-oil.html
- Broccoli Nutrition Facts. http://www.nutrition-and-you.com/broccoli.html
- Thiel, S. (2011). About Broccoli's Nutritional Value. http://www.livestrong.com/article/386500-about-broccolis-nutritional-values/
- Broccoli: The Crown Jewel of Nutrition. http://www.vegparadise.com/highestperch44.html
- The Benefits of Spinach Consumption. http://www.naturally-healthy-eating.com/benefits-of-spinach.html
- 11 Health Benefits of Spinach. http://www.healthdiaries.com/eatthis/11-health-benefits-of-spinach.html
- Magee, E. Health Properties of Tomatoes. http://www.webmd.com/food-recipes/features/health-properties-tomatoes
- 5 Health Benefits of Tomatoes. http://www.fitday.com/fitness-articles/nutrition/healthy-eating/5-health-benefits-of-tomatoes.html
- Cale, E.(2011). Sweet Potatoes and an Anti-Inflammatory Diet. http://www.livestrong.com/article/542069-sweet-potatoes-an-anti-inflammatory-diet/
- What's New and Beneficial about Sweet Potatoes. http://www.whfoods.com/genpage.php?tname=foodspice&dbid=64
- Bell pepper nutrition facts. http://www.nutrition-and-you.com/bell-pepper.html
- Bell Peppers. http://www.whfoods.com/genpage.php?tname=foodspice&dbid=50

- Lupton, J.R. (20120. From Basic Science to Dietary Guidance: Dietary Fiber as an Example. Journal of Food and Drug Analysis, Vol. 20, Suppl. 1, 2012, Pages 346
- Kerns, M. Nutrients Found in Figs. http://healthyeating.sfgate.com/nutrients-found-figs-2427.html
- Nutrients in Figs. http://www.whfoods.com/genpage.php?tname=foodspice&dbid=24
- Blueberries. http://www.whfoods.com/genpage.php?tname=foodspice&dbid=8
- Top 10 Health Benefits of Blueberries. http://www.womenfitness.net/blueberries.htm
- Kerri-Ann Jennings (2011). 6 Serious Health Benefits Of Apples: http://www.huffingtonpost.com/eatingwell/health-benefits-of-apples_b_966110.html#s364108&title=Nutrition_Straight_Up
- Apples—Overview. http://www.superfoodsrx.com/superfoods/apples/
- Doheny, K. (2012). Choose Dark Chocolate for Health Benefits. http://www.webmd.com/diet/news/20120424/pick-dark-chocolate-health-benefits
- Is Chocolate Good for Your Heart? http://my.clevelandclinic.org/heart/prevention/nutrition/chocolate.aspx
- What Are the Benefits of Asian Pears? http://www.livestrong.com/article/262437-what-are-the-benefits-of-asian-pears/
- Pears. http://www.whfoods.com/genpage.php?tname=foodspice&dbid=28
- Asian Pear Nutritional Information. http://www.livestrong.com/article/268152-asian-pear-nutritional-information/
- Lychee a Small But Powerful Berry. http://www.engineeredlifestyles.org/lychee.html
- Appleby, M. The Benefits of Lychee. http://healthyeating.sfgate.com/benefits-lychee-4480.html

- Stein,N. Is Guava Good for Your Heart?
  http://healthyeating.sfgate.com/guava-good-heart-1893.html
- Alternative Medicine: The Health and Medicinal Benefits of Guavas.
  http://www.oohoi.com/natural%20remedy/everyday_food/guava-health-benefits.htm
- McGee, E. The Secret of Edamame.
  http://www.webmd.com/diet/features/the-secret-of-edamame.
- Hackett, J. Tofu Nutritional Value Information.
  http://vegetarian.about.com/od/healthnutrition/p/tofunutrition.htm

4) Kettlebells for Dummies, Sarah Lurie, Wiley Publishing Inc.